NURSING

Nadia R. Singh, BSN, RN, is a registered nurse practicing in a medical oncology unit at the Jupiter Medical Center, Jupiter, Florida. Prior to this, she worked as a medical–surgical nurse in Boston, Massachusetts, and Florida. She is certified in IV infusion, telemetry, and pressure ulcer care (ANA), and in BLS/ACLS by the American Red Cross, and she is licensed to practice in Massachusetts, New York, and Florida. Ms. Singh graduated in 2008 with a bachelor of science in nursing (BSN) from Simmons College School of Nursing in Boston, Massachusetts, and is currently working toward her master's degree in nursing (MSN). She speaks to new nursing students at universities throughout southern Florida.

NURSING
The Ultimate Study Guide

Second Edition

Nadia R. Singh, BSN, RN

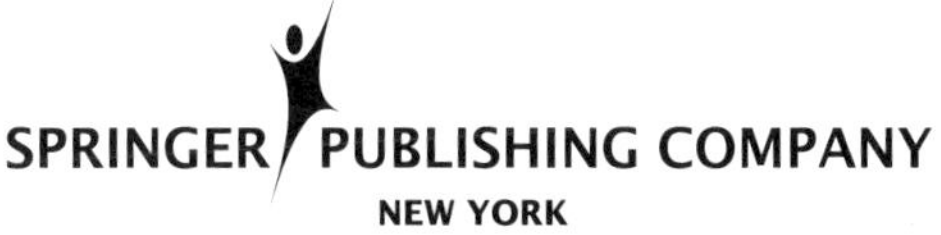

Springer Publishing Company, LLC
11 West 42nd Street
New York, NY 10036
www.springerpub.com

Acquisitions Editor: Elizabeth Nieginski
Production Editor: Kris Parrish
Composition: S4Carlisle Publishing Services

ISBN: 978-0-8261-3022-8
e-book ISBN: 978-0-8261-3023-5

15 16 17 18 / 5 4 3 2 1

Library of Congress Cataloging-in-Publication Data
Singh, Nadia R., author.
Nursing : the ultimate study guide / Nadia Singh.—Second edition.
p. ; cm.
Includes bibliographical references and index.
ISBN 978-0-8261-3022-8—ISBN 978-0-8261-3023-5 (e-book)
I. Title.
[DNLM: 1. Nursing Care. 2. Nursing. WY 100.1]
RT51
610.73—dc23

2015009944

Printed in the United States of America by McNaughton & Gunn.

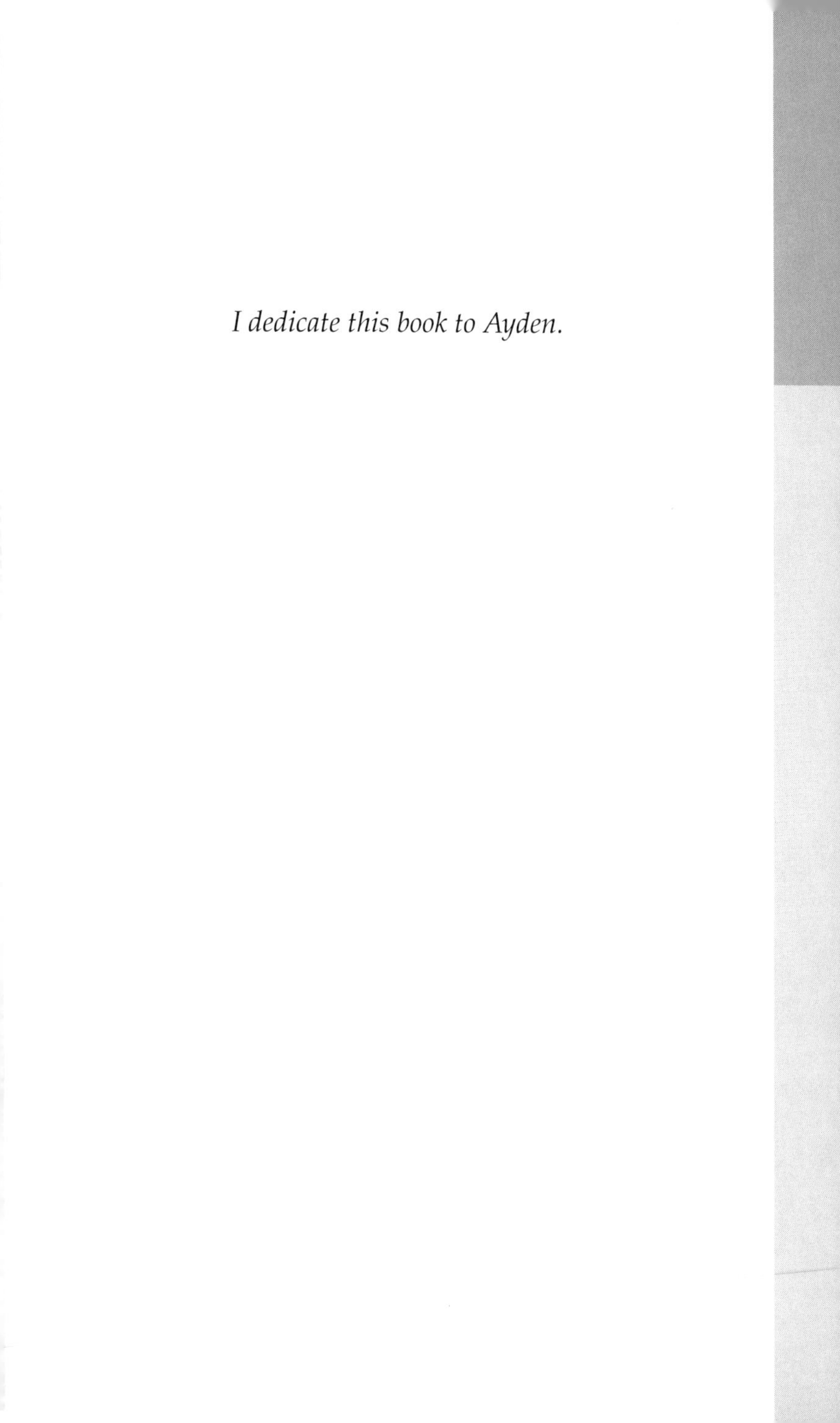

I dedicate this book to Ayden.

CONTENTS

PREFACE

In this second edition of *Nursing: The Ultimate Study Guide*, my goal is to continue to help students succeed in their nursing program. In this edition, I provide the most up-to-date information for each nursing course, with three new chapters—"What to Expect in Nursing School," "Decreasing Test Anxiety," and "Emergency Nursing." The medical field is continually changing; every year medications and lab values are updated, and new disorders or viruses identified. Providing students with the most up-to-date information is key to helping them succeed in their nursing studies.

As a recent graduate, I know how difficult and stressful the nursing program can be. Long nights, difficult tests, clinicals, and the struggle to maintain a social life can feel like an overwhelming burden. The intention of this study guide is to provide you with the most frequently tested information based on my experience, class notes, and previous exams. There is an abundance of information to learn in a short time; use your textbooks and class notes along with this study guide to help you.

The format of this study guide is simple, short, and to the point—a tiny study guide with a big punch. Each chapter represents a nursing course, with highlighted information and flags in the margin identifying the most frequently tested information. Chapters are short and to the point and, in contrast to many other study guides, highlight only the most important and tested information. Do not be surprised by the short chapters; each one is packed with useful information in an easy-to-read format. This study guide can be used from the first course, fundamentals of nursing, to the last course, which is helping you prepare for the NCLEX.

Nursing programs are difficult, but with hard work and a positive attitude, you will graduate and become a great nurse. Be proud of yourself: Nursing is one of the most rewarding jobs. You have been accepted into a nursing program, which is the first big step, and that is a huge accomplishment! This book will help you through your nursing program to further your accomplishments, giving you tips for test taking and preparing you for the NCLEX. I will also share some personal stories of my experience in a nursing program. So grab some coffee, go to a comfy study spot, and let's get started! Welcome to the world of nursing!

ACKNOWLEDGMENTS

First, I would like to acknowledge my family for all their love and support: my mom, Shabbena Singh, who continues to this day to support me in my nursing career; my father, Wayne Singh, for opening the doors of opportunity that contributed to my success; Asiff, for giving me all of his love and support while I was writing this book; and Ayden, my joy, who never stops smiling.

Simmons College, thank you for the education and the foundation that helped me create this study guide and become the nurse I am today.

To the staff at Springer Publishing Company, thank you for believing in this book and for all your help with editing, publication, and creativity. I am especially thankful to Margaret Zuccarini and Elizabeth Nieginski for believing in me and this book.

To the nurses and fellow coworkers, who continue to educate and help me grow in the field of nursing, I am so thankful! To all the nurses in the field, you are greatly appreciated, and those whose lives you have changed will never forget you.

ONE

FUNDAMENTALS OF NURSING

Welcome to the beginning of your nursing education! Fundamentals of Nursing is the first nursing class you will take to begin the nursing program. The skills you learn in this course will provide the foundation for the many nursing responsibilities you will assume throughout your career as both a nurse and a student. As you review the syllabus for this course, you might say to yourself, "OMG, how on earth am I supposed to learn all of this in a semester." Stay calm and take it one day (and one section) at a time. It will take some time to adjust to the demands of the nursing program. Over time, you will develop study skills and confidence, and before you know it, you will be a pro at studying.

Let's chat a little about what this course is all about. Fundamentals of nursing introduces you to the thorough assessment of patients, the nursing process, communication between nurse and patient, cultural differences, functional health patterns, and the overall framework of nursing practice. Think of it this way: When you build a house, you start with the foundation and then move to the framework, walls, and so on. I think you get the point. This class is the foundation for nursing, the beginning point. It gives you an overview of what to expect when working as a nurse.

It will take some time to learn the skills needed to assess patients; do not feel discouraged if you do not grasp the concepts right away. I found myself struggling at the beginning of the course. I felt overwhelmed, my mind was on overload from all the information, and I was nervous about performing the assessments in front of my classmates. I was not one for failure, but boy, did I feel like one at the beginning of this class. My test scores were poor, and my nervousness was undermining my assessment skills. I began to change my thinking. I studied day and night, went to study groups, and my grades began to improve. It is like the old saying: "Hard work does pay off." I developed my study skills during this course, which helped me through the other courses, as well. You, too, will develop and improve your study skills as you progress through the course. So let's jump to it and get started! We will begin with the history of nursing.

HISTORY OF NURSING

We could talk all day about the history of nursing. Many books have been written describing the great works of the nurses who built the foundation for the nursing profession. Without their knowledge and perseverance, we would not have the growing field we do today. This chapter covers only a few details from the history of nursing. To be honest, very little of this historical information was tested, and I would not spend too much time trying to remember dates and exact timelines. Follow your professors' key points and highlight any information they emphasize. You will be required to know the influence of Florence Nightingale and her role in nursing.

→ • **Florence Nightingale laid the foundation for professional nursing practice through her work in the Crimea in the 1850s. She later established her own nursing school.** Through her teaching and emphasis on sanitary care of patients, the nursing field progressed.
- Nightingale was the first nurse epidemiologist.
- The Civil War (1860–1865) furthered the expansion of the nursing field. Nurses were needed to tend to patients' wounds, and the field began to grow as additional women were trained. It was also during this time that the American Red Cross was founded.
- Between 1860 and 1900, Nightingale established 400 nursing training schools and helped improve the conditions of hospital-based care.
- In 1956, the first Health Amendment Act gave nurses the financial aid needed for training and school.

This short outline summarizes the points to focus on when studying nursing history. The most frequently tested information was on Florence Nightingale and her influence. Refer to your classroom notes and what the professor highlights for more in-depth information. The following chapters will focus directly on patient care and assessments.

THERAPEUTIC COMMUNICATION

E-mails, text messages, Instagram, Facebook, WhatsApp, and Twitter are all forms of communication that we use in our daily lives. When communicating one on one with a patient, we must use compassion and care. Also, take into consideration the age and culture of the patients. It is unlikely that your 88-year-old patient will know the new lingo of "LOL" or "OMG." However, this may be just what is needed to connect with your younger patients. Communication in nursing is so important. Patients and families are often scared or worried, and you are often their source of information and comfort. When entering a patient's room, smile and introduce yourself to both the patient and the patient's family. Make them feel comfortable and well taken care of.

There are two types of communication: (a) verbal, which involves speaking to the patient, and (b) nonverbal, which involves the use of facial expressions, eye contact, and therapeutic touch. Remember, culture also plays a role in communication, which will be discussed in further detail in the next section.

Phases of Communication

There are three basic phases of communication: (a) introductory, (b) working, and (c) termination. You will use these three phases to understand your patient's problems and come up with solutions. In the *introductory phase,* you will introduce yourself, discuss any problems, and establish a relationship with your patient. Remember not every patient is cheery and upbeat. You will also have patients who are scared, angry, or discouraged. It will be your job to think of ways to establish an amicable relationship. Also, if a language barrier is present, this would be the best time to contact a translator.

The *working phase* is where you identify the patient's problem. For example, suppose the patient diagnosis is abdominal pain. In this phase, you would look further into why the patient is having abdominal pain using labs, scans, or physician notes. You would look for any resolution to the problems. Did the doctor prescribe pain medications? Was a CT scan performed? Is surgery necessary? The working phase is where the problem is identified and measures are taken to help the patient.

The last phase, the *termination phase,* is where the problem is being resolved. In the preceding example, if the patient was given pain medication as ordered and the problem has resolved, the nurse's communication with the patient would come to an end.

When thinking about the phases of communication, consider how you communicate when chatting with a friend, family member, or coworker who has a problem. They call you and state their problem. You talk about the problem and figure out ways to make it better. By the end of the conversation, your friend feels better because a resolution has been achieved or is in the making. Similarly, your patients are talking with you in the role of their problem solver, the one who makes them better. For all of you nervous nellies who are uncomfortable speaking with people, now is the time to practice and muster up some confidence. Communication is the key to nursing; it involves constant talking with patients, families, and physicians.

Tips on What *Not* to Do During Communication

When communicating with patients, there are some pitfalls you need to avoid. Do not be judgmental or abrupt, or speak down to patients. Avoid leading questions that may discourage or embarrass the patient. Do not crack jokes or speak about topics that may cause a patient to become offended. If language barriers are present, do not ignore these patients because you cannot understand them: Use an interpreter to communicate with the patient and try to avoid using family members to translate.

Developing Communication Skills

There are several ways to create a great relationship with patients. Most important is to provide privacy when speaking with the patient—for example, by closing the door or shutting the curtain. Introducing yourself is the next step. Sit down, if possible, when talking—patients feel more comfortable when you are speaking to them at eye level. Listen carefully, and strive to make a comfortable environment for the patient.

→ **Use open-ended questions. Avoid yes/no answers to encourage your patients to give you details when discussing their health problems. You want as much information as possible, including anything about their past medical history.**

Be compassionate. Being in the hospital is scary for both patients and families. Emotional support is often needed. For patients who are confused or unable to respond, the use of touch is therapeutic. As a nurse, you will create ways of your own to make communication comfortable for you and the patient.

THE NURSING PROCESS (NURSING CARE PLANS)

Along with communication techniques, nurses rely on the nursing process when caring for patients. The nursing process is a five-step systematic approach to problem solving. It allows the nurse to obtain both subjective and objective information to determine the health care problem. The five steps are (a) *a*ssessment, (b) *d*iagnosis, (c) *p*lanning, (d) *i*mplementation, and (e) *e*valuation, which can be remembered using the mnemonic "ADPIE (A Delicious PIE)." Based on these steps a care plan is conducted for each patient.

Assessment

Begin your assessment by asking the patient about the problem, signs, and symptoms that he or she has been experiencing. If the patient is unable to speak, ask a family member if present what has been going on with the patient. During an assessment, two types of data are obtained: *subjective* and *objective*. Subjective data are symptoms that the patient describes to you (e.g., "My arm feels itchy and has little red bumps all over" or "I feel like there is a ton of bricks sitting on my chest.") Objective data are findings that are observed, assessed, and documented by the nurse (e.g., "There is a quarter size rash located on the right arm with redness" or "The patient's respirations are increasing, and he is huddled over in pain.") **Objective data are any signs that can be observed, and vital signs are a type of objective data.** ←

The first step is to assess the areas that can help you formulate a diagnosis. A patient can have numerous problems that can result in more than one diagnosis. For instance, a patient may have high blood pressure and a constant headache. The diagnosis would be hypertension and pain. Information can be obtained from the patient, medical records, family members, and physical examination.

Diagnosis

A diagnosis is obtained on the basis of the patient's assessment findings. A *nursing diagnosis* is the statement of a problem based on the actual signs and symptoms the patient is experiencing. For example, consider a patient who is admitted with pneumonia. One diagnosis for this patient might be "ineffective airway clearance related to accumulation of secretions." This diagnosis indicates that patient is experiencing shortness of breath due to a productive cough. In simple terms, the nursing diagnosis is the statement of the patient's problems and the causes.

During your clinical experience, your professor will ask you to compile a list of nursing diagnoses based on the patient you have assessed. Typically, two or three nursing diagnoses are requested. This would be a great time to invest in a nursing diagnosis book to familiarize yourself with these types of diagnostic statements. Diagnosing the patient will help with planning care for this particular patient and will help you focus on the problems at hand.

Planning

Once the nursing diagnoses are obtained, it is time to start planning patient care and interventions. Based on the diagnoses, the next step is to formulate goals and outcomes for the patient. For example, take the patient who was admitted with pneumonia. The nursing diagnosis is ineffective airway clearance related to accumulation of secretions. The corresponding nursing interventions are to perform chest physiotherapy to help loosen and bring up the secretions, to elevate the head of the bed to aid breathing, and to obtain the oxygen saturation level every hour. The nursing interventions are what you as a nurse can do to help the patient.

Implementation

Once the patient is assessed, the diagnoses are made, and the planning is in place, you are ready to implement the steps of the nursing care plan. It is important to establish a realistic time frame for the patient to meet the identified goals and interventions. In this section of the care plan, you should provide scientific rationales to explain your diagnoses in further detail. Refer to your textbook and online resources for all scientific rationales. You should have a rationale for each intervention. For example, for the patient with pneumonia, the scientific rationale for patient positioning is that an upright position facilitates normal anatomical position and allows greater lung expansion for proper oxygen exchange. This gives support to the diagnosis based on facts and research.

Evaluation

We have arrived at the last step in the ladder of "ADPIE"! This is the completion of the nursing care plan. The patient has been assessed and diagnosed, planning is in place, implementation is complete, and evaluation of the patient's response to these actions is underway. It is during this step that the patient goals are met or close to being met as a result of nursing interventions.

The nursing process is important in patient care. It is a system to help nurses identify patient problems and, along with doctors, develop a plan to help the patient. You will use this process in nursing school and as a nurse. It is an essential part of patient care and recovery. It is not important to memorize each approved nursing diagnosis; you will not be tested on your knowledge of each one. Instead, use your nursing diagnosis book to help you as you construct your patient care plan.

PATIENT EDUCATION

From the time a patient is first admitted up to the day of discharge, patient education is very important. It is important for the patient to know and be aware of nursing care each step of the way. Explain patients' medical diagnoses and provide printouts for them to review and read. Obtain information on any allergies. Explain each medication and make sure patients have a proper understanding of what it does and how it is going to help them. Maintain privacy and follow HIPAA guidelines when educating patients and families. Patients and their families feel most comfortable when they know what is going on and why. Discharge education is important to provide patients with the information needed for self-care at home. The information you provide to patients can help them on their journey to recovery at home. Most institutes provide materials for patients that you can print out and provide during their hospital stay and upon discharge.

CARE ACROSS A LIFE SPAN

Infant (birth–1 year)	• Infants react to sound and voices. They gain 5–7 ounces per week. They gain head control and begin to roll. • Maintain safety. Follow a feeding schedule. Follow up with immunizations. Maintain a healthy sleep schedule.
Toddler (1–3 years)	• Toddlers start to crawl, then walk. They begin to explore and touch. They begin to eat solid food and use utensils. They begin to talk and learn. • Maintain safety. Use gates for kitchens and stairs. Do not leave small objects on the floor; toddlers have a tendency to place everything in their mouths.
Preschool (3–5 years)	• Preschool children begin to ride bikes and run in the playground. They love to use their imaginations. They begin to learn the alphabet and are able to form sentences. • Start teaching safety measures such as wearing helmets.
School-age child (6–10 years)	• School-age children begin to gain independence. They are adventurous. • Maintain a schedule and hygiene, and initiate rules. Minimize fears. Teach safety measures. Maintain immunizations.

Adolescents (11–17 years)	• Adolescents begin to have independence. They start driving and going out with friends. • Initiate limits and rules. Teach adolescents to avoid smoking, drugs, and alcohol. Teach about safe sex and pregnancy prevention. Encourage positive behavior. Monitor for bullying and depression.
Young adult (18–30 years)	Young adults have reached full maturity. They begin to work regularly and start careers. They feel confident in making choices. They begin to have families.
Adult (30–60 years)	Health begins to decline. Adults begin to care for their parents as they age. Family responsibilities increase. Stress tends to increase.
Older adult (60+ years)	Health problems increase. Retirement takes place. Older adults may enter an assisted living facility. Help with activities of daily living may be needed. Older adults may struggle with aging. Safety for older adults may need to be improved, especially those experiencing forgetfulness or confusion.

FUNCTIONAL HEALTH PATTERNS

Functional health patterns are the basis for a series of questions that the nurse asks the patient to develop an in-depth nursing assessment. These questions help the nurse gain a better idea of the patient's overall health and lifestyle. They are part of the admission process when a patient is admitted to the hospital. The functional health patterns encompass the patient's general health, nutrition, elimination, activity, sleep, cognition, living environment, abuse, sexuality, spiritual/cultural beliefs, coping mechanisms, hygiene, and self-perception. They give the nurses and team a better understanding of the patient's situation in order to address problems and develop a plan for proper care, planning, and safety. It's like my mom used to say, "If you don't ask, you won't know!" It is important to maintain patient privacy while asking about these topics. If family members are present, you may want to ask them to step out of the room while these questions are asked.

I am warning you, as you review your packet of health patterns and the questions that are asked, that not all of the topics covered by these questions will be comfortable ones for you to discuss. I have to admit that, as a nursing student and as a nurse, I would blush when discussing sexuality with my 80- or 90-year-old patients. Most would reply, "Great, that's why

I take Viagra." Never a dull moment in nursing, I will tell you that! Now I will not go into depth on each health pattern. Refer to your packet or book for the questions that should be asked. Again, you will not be tested on your knowledge of each question; rather, the goal is to become familiar with the health patterns and to become comfortable obtaining the information from patients during your assessment.

CULTURAL DIFFERENCES

As a nurse and student, it is important to be aware of the cultural diversity among patients. It is important to identify and respect each patient's culture, religion, and beliefs. When obtaining a patient's past medical history, you should ask about and identify any spiritual or cultural beliefs. If there is a language barrier, use the interpreter services provided by your hospital or facility for assistance. Here are some important and common cultural beliefs to remember:

- In many Asian cultures, making direct eye contact can be offensive.
- In the Muslim religion, pork and pork products are prohibited.
- People who practice as Jehovah's Witnesses do not receive blood products.
- For many cultures, in the interest of modesty, men are not allowed to be the caretakers of women; in these cases, a woman caretaker is preferred.

NUTRITION

It is important to monitor the intake and output of all patients, making sure that patients have the correct amount of calories for their weight. A diet will be ordered for your patient based on his or her condition and medical history. For example, a patient who is admitted with cardiac complications will receive what is called a cardiac diet, which is low in sodium and fat. Patients who are malnourished will be placed on a high-calorie diet and may need IV nutrition. Also, pay attention to any cultural preferences that may be needed for a patient's diet. Listed here are some common diets you will see ordered:

- Regular diet: There are no restrictions to diet or calories.
- Cardiac diet: For cardiac patients, includes food low in sodium and fat.
- Clear/full liquid: Ordered for patients before any GI diagnostics or after surgery. Clear liquid includes anything clear

such as apple juice, tea, broth, popsicles, ginger ale, or Sprite. → **Avoid any liquids that are flavored or colored red for patients with gastrointestinal bleeds.** Full liquids include liquid foods; there are no restrictions.

- Soft/mechanical soft diets: These consist of foods that are easy to swallow and chew. Mechanical soft include mashed potatoes, ground meats, and other easy-to-swallow foods.
- Renal diet: These consist of foods that are low in sodium and potassium. Protein intake is also monitored.
- When monitoring a patient's nutrition, also be aware of any precautions such as those required for patients who are at risk for aspiration or who have difficulty chewing. Assist patients who need to be fed, as well. It is the nurse's responsibility to assess for any changes in feeding ability and nutritional status.

URINARY AND BOWEL FUNCTION

Assessing a patient's intake and output is very important. Most physicians will order strict intake and output on patients, especially surgical or renal patients. It is the nurse's responsibility to make sure that the patient is urinating and having regular bowel movements every shift or daily. There are various reasons why a patient's urinary or bowel elimination may be disrupted. For example, renal patients who are on dialysis are anuric (or have little output). It is important to monitor any patient who has not had a bowel movement for several days as this may indicate a small bowel obstruction or severe constipation. During your assessment, it is important to ask the patient whether he or she is urinating regularly and having regular bowel movements. Remember, each patient is different; ask your patients what their normal habits are.

Urinary Elimination

→ **An adult patient's urinary output should total at least 30 mL every hour.** This is measured by asking the patient to void in a plastic container that is placed in the toilet for accurate measurement; if the patient has a Foley catheter, the measurement is taken from the Foley drainage bag. Males may use urinals to measure accurate output. It is important to look at the urine; normal urine is yellow and clear. The presence of blood in the urine or cloudy or foul-smelling urine can signify a urinary problem or infection. A Foley catheter may be ordered for various reasons. Surgical, urinary incontinence, ICU patients, and others may require a Foley catheter during their hospital stay. Refer to your class notes and visual images in your textbook on how to insert a Foley catheter. (I could write the procedure out for you, but, to be honest, you really need a visual picture in order to understand it.) Common urinary complications that can occur are:

- Urinary tract infection (UTI): An infection in the urinary tract that causes burning during urination, hematuria, foul-smelling urine. Elderly patients who present with a UTI may have confusion as an associated symptom.
- Incontinence: A person's inability to control the function of urination. In many cases, briefs are worn to prevent urinary leakage.

Bowel Elimination

This topic and discussing a patient's bowel movements may not be the highlight of your day. But it is important to ask patients if they are having daily movements and making sure they are staying regular. Although it is not always necessary to assess the stool, complications can arise for which you will have to obtain a specimen or check the stool. Common bowel complications are:

- Constipation: The inability to have a bowel movement. Stool softeners, prune juice, or laxatives may be given to promote bowel movements. Common causes of constipation are pain medications, immobility, or bowel obstruction.
- Occult stool: Blood in the stool caused by various conditions such as hemorrhoids or ulcers.
- Diarrhea: Loose bowel movements that vary in severity. Can be caused by medications, food poisoning, viruses, and bacteria such as *Clostridium difficile* (*C. diff*).

VITAL SIGNS

Vital signs, by definition, are a person's temperature, pulse/heart rate (HR), respiration rate, blood pressure (BP), and pain level. A person's vital signs reflects his or her respiratory function, cardiac stability, and hemodynamic status. Changes in vital signs can indicate disorders such as hypertension (high BP), hypotension (low BP), dehydration, respiratory distress, hypoxemia (low O_2 levels), tachycardia (increased pulse), and bradycardia (low HR). You will need to become familiar with these signs and practice obtaining accurate results. You will have plenty of time to practice on other students and those good-looking mannequins in the lab. At the end of the semester, you will go to the hospital or nursing home to practice on patients.

Time for a funny story that I know some of you will relate to. I had almost completed my fundamentals course and was at a local nursing home assessing a patient's vital signs. I felt comfortable and confident because I thought I had this skill down pat. When I exited the room, one of the nurses on the floor walked up and asked, "Did you take his temperature with the red thermometer?" My response, with hesitation, was yes. She chuckled a little and said, "Well, those red thermometers are used only for rectal temperatures." I was mortified, even though the thermometer was clean and capped. I was thinking to myself that it would have been nice if someone had told me. My confidence level went from 100% to 0% in no time. It is true that we learn from our mistakes, because I never made that mistake again. So always remember when you see a red thermometer, red stands for "rectal." With that said, let's go on to describe each vital sign.

Body Temperature

Definition: A measurement of the body's temperature in degrees. **The body's temperature is controlled by the hypothalamus. This is in the preoptic part of the brain.** The hypothalamus is able to detect when the body's temperature is too high, indicating a fever, or too low, indicating hypothermia. A normal temperature on average is about 98.6°F (36°C).

Assessing the Temperature: The four main ways to assess body temperature are (a) oral, (b) rectal (most reliable), (c) axillary (under the arms), and (d) tympanic. Many hospitals use an electronic thermometer to obtain oral temperature readings. **Never use a rectal temperature on patients who are immunocompromised (have reduced immune function). When obtaining an oral temperature, make sure that the patient has not had anything hot or cold to drink for 15 minutes before the assessment, as this can alter the temperature.** It is important to tell your instructor or the nurse about any changes in a patient's temperature.

Factors That Affect Temperature: Age, exercise, stress, illness, and infection can all affect the temperature.

Temperature Gone Wrong: Changes can occur, and these are defined as pyrexia, hyperpyrexia, and hypothermia. In reality, nurses just say, "The temperature is high." But it is important to know these terms. Pyrexia means an elevation in temperature, hyperpyrexia means a critical increase in temperature, and hypothermia is a temperature lower than average.

Pulse

Definition: When the left ventricle pumps blood through the heart, it causes a pulse. **The heart pumps about 5 L of blood per minute.** This would be a great time to look over your anatomy and physiology book to review the structures and functioning of the heart. Remember the term *cardiac output;* this is the term used to describe the amount of blood pumped each minute through the circulatory system. The normal adult pulse ranges from 60 to 100 beats per minute (bpm).

Assessing the Pulse: The pulse can be obtained from various parts of the body. Most commonly used is the radial pulse found on the wrist. You can auscultate (listen to the pulse with a stethoscope), palpate (feel the pulse), or use a Doppler stethoscope to hear the pulse as well. During an assessment, you will have to obtain a pulse from various sites on the body. **The apical pulse is located between the fourth and fifth left intercostal space; it is the strongest pulse in the body and provides an accurate indication of the HR.** The radial pulse is located at the wrist right below the thumb (most commonly assessed). The brachial pulse is in the pit of the arm, known as the antecubital fossa. Carotid pulses are on the side of the neck. Femoral pulses are in a part the groin known as the inguinal area. The pedal pulses are along the top of the foot, in between the big toe and the second toe.

Factors That Affect Pulse: Age, gender, exercise, medications, stress, anxiety, positional changes, illness, and blood loss can alter pulse rates. Infants have a higher pulse rate of 110 to 160 bpm. School-age children have pulse rates of 75 to 120 bpm on average. Take age into consideration when obtaining a pulse.

Pulse Gone Wrong: An electrocardiogram (EKG) is used to determine a person's cardiac rhythm and HR. Normal sinus rhythm means the patient has a normal rate and rhythm. Dysrhythmia is a change in the heart's rhythm or pulse pattern. An increase in the HR (above 100) is termed tachycardia, and a decrease in the HR (below 60) is termed bradycardia. Many changes in rhythm can occur; these are described in further detail in Chapter 3. Patients are often placed on cardiac monitors or telemetry to monitor irregular pulses or heart rhythms.

Respirations

Definition: Gas exchange is the exchange of carbon dioxide with oxygen in the lungs. It is the body's way of regulating oxygen through the circulatory system to maintain healthy cells through inspiration and exhalation. Here is a little exercise: Take a deep breath in; this is called inspiration. Now breathe out; this is called exhalation. A normal respiratory rate is 16 to 20 breaths *per minute.*

Assessing Respirations: The first step is to assess the patient. Is the patient breathing normally? Is the patient having difficulty breathing? Are the breaths shallow? Is there use of accessory muscles in breathing? These can all be assessed by looking at the patient and listening to his or her lungs. You can also ask the patient for a past medical history of respiratory problems, such as asthma, or inquire whether he or she smokes, because that can affect respiration. After a visual assessment, auscultate, or listen to the patient's lungs by placing the stethoscope on the upper chest and lower chest and counting the breaths per minute. → **An easy way to determine the respiration rate is by counting the number of breaths for 30 seconds and then multiplying by 2 to get a full minute rate.** Have the patient sit upright and instruct the patient not to speak during the assessment.

Factors That Affect Respirations: Smoking, stress, anxiety, exercise, temperature, infection, pneumonia, asthma, underlying physiological causes, and medications affect respiration. There are a lot more factors that can change a patient's respiration, but these are the most common. I am going to share with you the biggest nursing secret of all time: → **During an exam, when you are asked a priority question such as which patient to see first, always choose the answer that refers to a patient with a compromised respiratory system! Choose answers that coincide with the "ABCs" (airway, breathing, and circulation). Always help the patient who is in respiratory distress first.**

Respirations Gone Wrong: An increase in respirations is referred to as tachypnea (anything greater than 20 breaths per minute). A decrease in respirations is referred to as bradypnea (less than 12 breaths per minute). → **Remember any words that have the ending –pnea refer to a change in respirations.** I know all this information seems like a lot to remember; take a deep breath so you don't experience any respiratory changes.

Blood Pressure

Definition: Blood pressure (BP) is the force of blood against the walls of the blood vessels, especially the arteries. Picture a waterslide of blood pushing against the artery walls, creating pressure. Two terms are used to describe BP: *diastolic* and *systolic*. A normal BP is anything below 120/80 mmHg. The systolic number, 120 mmHg, indicates the pressure in the circulatory system during the contraction of the heart. The diastolic number, 80 mmHg, is the pressure when the heart is at rest or relaxation.

Assessing the Blood Pressure: Blood pressure is obtained by using a BP cuff, also known as a sphygmomanometer (try saying that three times fast), and a stethoscope. There should be a picture of this device in your class notes or textbook. ← **The part of the cuff that goes around the patient's upper arm should be placed over two-thirds of the length of the upper arm and cover three-fourths of the circumference of the arm, right above the antecubital fossa (middle part of the arm).** The sounds that are heard are called Korotkoff sounds, which can also be visualized on the meter and represent the systolic and diastolic pressures. When the cuff is inflated, the strongest beat will represent the systolic pressure, usually at 120 mmHg, and the deflation of the cuff and the last beat seen on the meter will be the diastolic pressure, at 80 mmHg. When measuring a patient's BP, use the correct size of cuff for the arm; some patients may require a small cuff. BP should not be taken on the arm on the same side where patients have undergone a mastectomy or where a peripherally inserted central catheter (PICC) line is inserted. Do not leave the cuff inflated as this can cause discomfort. Make sure the BP is taken on the bare skin and not over clothing. If there is a significant change in BP on the electronic cuff, a manual reading is performed through auscultation. Any changes in BP must be reported.

Factors That Affect Blood Pressure: Factors that affect BP are dehydration, stress, medications, illness, surgery, hemorrhage, and pain.

Blood Pressure Gone Wrong: A BP greater than 120/80 mmHg is hypertensive. A BP below 120/80 mmHg is hypotensive. Orthostatic hypotension is a decrease in blood pressure that occurs when patients change from a lying position to a standing position. ← **If a patient is orthostatic, make sure you help them to stand, as a loss of balance or dizziness may occur.** Hypertension and hypotension are discussed in further detail in Chapter 3.

This completes an overview of the vital signs in a nutshell. In hospitals, an electronic Dynamap machine is used to obtain vital signs. It is important to memorize and identify any changes in vital signs and report them immediately. They are called "vital" for a reason: The changes in these signs are usually the first signs that something is wrong in a patient.

Pain

Pain is sometimes referred to as the fifth vital sign. Use a numeric pain scale to identify the patient's pain level. Pain can signify that something is wrong; therefore it is important to identify and treat at once. Pain can be acute or chronic. Medicate pain as prescribed. It is important to maintain comfort for the patient and assess pain throughout the shift. Pain medications are ordered based on the patient's diagnosis and severity. There are five major types of pain:

- Acute pain: New onset, lasting a short time and usually affecting one area.
- Chronic pain: Experienced over a long period of time; it is constant and persistent.
- Neuropathic pain: Caused by damage to the peripheral nerves.
- Phantom pain: Postamputation, patient can feel pain in the extremity.
- Nociceptive pain: Pain in the muscles or joints.

Methods of pain relief may include medications, relaxation, and touch. Pain medications ordered can be narcotics or nonnarcotic analgesics. A PCA (patient-controlled analgesic) may be ordered for patients postoperatively to better control pain. It is important to identify where the patient is having pain, have the patient use either the numeric or the FLACC (Face, Legs, Activity, Cry, Consolability) scale to rate the pain, and document.

SKIN INTEGRITY AND IMMOBILITY

Immobility is defined as the loss or lack of movement of the legs or arms or both. This can have various causes such as paralysis, bedridden patients who have lost the ability to walk, or surgical procedures that require the patient to stay in bed. When a patient is confined to one position, complications can arise. Complications such as pressure ulcers, blood clots, and contractures of the extremities are the most common. Nursing interventions for the immobile patient are:

- Turning and repositioning the patient every 2 hours
- Maintaining proper skin care; applying lotion or barrier cream to affected areas
- Ensuring proper hydration by increasing the patient's fluid intake and encouraging him or her to drink water, or through intravenous fluids
- Performing range of motion (ROM) to increase mobility and decrease the risk of contractures of the muscles
- A specialty mattress, such as an air mattress, may be ordered for the patient.
- A wound care consult may also be needed for complex wounds

Common Complications of Immobility

Ulcers

You will be responsible for memorizing and identifying the stages of skin breakdown and healing. Patients who are immobile, especially elderly patients, are at risk for pressure ulcers. A pressure ulcer is a sore that occurs in the skin, causing damage to various layers as a result of constant pressure exerted on one area of the body. **Pressure ulcers are classified into four stages based on severity. Refer to your textbook for a visual; you will be tested on the different stages.** Ulcers commonly occur on bony prominences such as the coccyx, heels, elbows, hips, and ankles. This is caused by shearing, tension, and friction on the skin. **As a nurse, your responsibility is to prevent pressure ulcers by repositioning the patient every 2 hours, applying barrier creams, maintaining dressing changes, and providing adequate hydration.** The four stages of pressure ulcers are:

Stage I: Reddening of the skin on the epidermal layer. Skin is intact.

Stage II: Reddening and edema of the epidermis and dermis layer. Similar to a blister. Skin is blanchable.

Stage III: Injury to the subcutaneous layer. Fat may be visible but bones, tendons, or muscles are not exposed.

Stage IV: Severe damage to all layers of the skin with exposed bone, tendon, or muscle.

A visual of these stages will give you a better understanding. A wound care consult may be needed. Dressings such as Duoderm or Aquacel may be needed. Refer to your class notes and your textbook for pictures of different positioning that is used for patients.

Deep Vein Thrombosis

Poor circulation and blood flow resulting from immobility can lead to thrombus formation in the veins and arteries. The most common place for a clot to develop is in the calf. Symptoms of a blood clot are warmth at the site, pain, swelling, and redness. An ultrasound is used to determine whether a clot is present. Patients who are immobile are placed on venous thromboembolism (VTE) prophylactics such as thromboembolism-deterrent (TED) compression stockings or a sequential compression device (SCD) to prevent blood clots. The patient may also be placed on an anticoagulant (blood thinner) such as heparin or Lovenox to decrease the risk for clots. → **Do not place SCDs or TEDS on the leg with blood clots; this can cause the clot to travel or move.** The key is anticoagulation is dissolving the clot before it moves through the vein or artery or becomes larger in size.

It is the nurse's responsibility to maintain skin integrity and avoid complications in the immobile patient. When taking care of elderly patients who are immobile, use careful measures when turning and repositioning due to fragile skin and weakness. Report any changes in skin to your instructor.

Wound Care

A part of maintaining skin integrity is performing proper wound care and dressing changes. It is important to examine and dress the wound based on the physician's orders. When a wound is present, you must first take a picture and obtain an exact measurement of the wound. It is important to maintain a clean and sterile environment for any open wounds. Once a sterile field is in place, clean the wound with either normal saline or sterile water, using gauze to clean in and around the wound bed. The type of dressing used will depend on the wound; the most common type is wet to dry. Check the doctor's orders to see if packing of the wound is needed. Packing involves inserting small strips of gauze, usually ¼ inch wide, into the wound. Cover the wound with a 4-inch by 4-inch gauze and tape. Use only sterile surgical equipment when changing a dressing. At times, the physician may order ointments such as Santyl (collagenase) to be applied to the wound bed for further treatment. A Duoderm or Aquacel dressing to be placed over the wound may also be ordered. When undressing a wound, throw away the old dressing in a red contamination bag, and change gloves when applying a clean dressing. Document that the new dressing was completed. In severe cases, a wound vac is used for continuous drainage of the wound through suction, which is used for a series of days and is only temporary.

OXYGENATION

Oxygenation involves the amount of oxygen flow to the tissues. I am going to let you in on a little secret, probably the most important piece of advice you will receive during nursing school: Assessing a patient's respiratory status is always a priority. When a patient is experiencing any respiratory abnormalities, difficulty breathing, shortness of breath, or labored breathing, you need to assess and treat immediately. **On exams and tests, when any questions have to do with assessing an airway or treating a patient who has difficulty breathing, the answer always is: Assess the airway first!** Oxygen saturation is used to determine the amount of oxygen perfusion through the body. The normal values are 96% to 100%. Keep in mind that a patient with a respiratory disorder may require oxygen. ←

Common Respiratory Disorders:

- Chronic obstructive pulmonary disease (COPD)
- Asthma
- Pneumonia/bronchitis

Alterations in Breathing Patterns

Normal respirations are usually 12 to 20 per minute.

- Tachypnea: A rapid increase in respirations to anything above 22 respirations per minute. It is caused by fever, asthma, hyperventilation, anxiety, or pain. Patients present with fast and labored breathing.
- Bradypnea: Slow respirations of less than 12 breaths per minute. It is caused by pain medication or happens when a patient is sleeping.
- Kussmaul breathing: Deep and rapid breaths are usually seen in patients who are experiencing metabolic acidosis (excess acid in the tissues) and can be caused by chronic kidney disease or diabetic ketoacidosis.
- Cheyne–Stokes breathing: Very deep and shallow breaths. Commonly seen in patients with congestive heart failure and in terminally ill patients, as well.

Respiratory Diagnostics

When a patient is experiencing a change in respiratory status, it is important to obtain the correct labs and exams to determine the cause. Diagnostics such as complete blood count (CBC), chest x-ray, arterial blood gases, pulse oximetry, sputum culture, computed tomography angiography (CTA) of the chest, and many others may be used to help diagnose and treat respiratory disorders.

Nursing Intervention

When a patient is experiencing a change in respiratory status, first assess the airway and oxygen saturation. Call for help from either the respiratory therapist or team on the floor. Call the doctor for orders. If the patient is experiencing shortness of breath, place the patient in semi-Fowler's position (an upright sitting position with the head of the bed elevated greater than 45°). Administer oxygen as ordered. **A nasal cannula is commonly used to supply oxygen to the patient. When placing the nasal cannula, set the amount to 2 L, and adjust it per physician's order.** In an emergency situation, the patient may require a mask that supplies a larger amount of oxygen.

There are nonemergent nursing interventions that you can perform to facilitate breathing without a physician's order. Chest physiotherapy (Chest PT) is used to break up secretion in the chest so the patient can better expel the secretions. This is performed by cupping the hands and beating gently on the patient's upper back. Giving the patient an incentive spirometer (IS) helps the patient expand the lungs and alveoli. Instructing the patient to take deep breaths and cough every 2 hours can help prevent hospital-acquired disorders such as pneumonia. Nebulizer treatments and steroids may also be needed for the patient.

An early sign of a lack of oxygen is a change in mental status and low oxygen saturation levels, and a late sign is clubbing of the nails.

ACID–BASE IMBALANCES

Oxygen saturation level is determined by arterial blood gas (ABG) results—in other words, the amount of oxygen that is flowing in the arteries. The acid–base levels are based on pH, CO_2, $PaCO_2$, O_2, PaO_2, HCO_3, and H. Changes in these levels cause acid–base imbalances. When a patient's respiratory status is impaired, ABGs must be obtained to determine accurate readings. ABGs can be obtained only by a physician or a respiratory therapist using what is called an Allen's test. I know this may be difficult to grasp at first, but with a little practice, you will be able to identify the imbalances. **It is important to know the**

normal values in order to identify the imbalance. Respiratory disorders such as COPD, asthma, or upper respiratory infections can cause imbalances.

Blood Gas Values:

- pH: 7.35–7.45
- $PaCO_2$: 35–45 mmHg
- PaO_2: 80–100 mmHg
- HCO_3: 22–26 mEq/L

Changes in Acid–Base Balance

Respiratory Acidosis

In this condition, $PaCO_2$ is increased above 45 mmHg and pH is decreased (below 7.45). Respiratory acidosis can be caused by obstructive pulmonary diseases, pneumonia, hypoventilation, and asthma. Symptoms are rapid/shallow respirations, confusion, and hypoxemia. **Nursing interventions are to maintain the patient's oxygen saturation levels and airway, and treat the underlying cause.** Mechanical ventilation may be needed.

Respiratory Alkalosis

In this condition, $PaCO_2$ is decreased and pH is increased. Respiratory alkalosis is caused by hyperventilation and stress. Symptoms are muscle twitching, deep/rapid breathing, dizziness, tingling of the fingers, and difficulty breathing. Nursing interventions treat the underlying cause and use a rebreathing mask.

Metabolic Acidosis

In this condition, both pH and HCO_3 are low. Metabolic acidosis is caused by renal failure, diarrhea, diabetes, vomiting, and shock. Symptoms are fruity breath, nausea, Kussmaul breathing, vomiting, diarrhea, headache, and increased potassium. **Nursing interventions are to administer intravenous sodium bicarbonate and maintain respiratory status.** Ensure proper nutrition and adequate hydration. **Monitor potassium levels.**

Metabolic Alkalosis

In this condition, pH and HCO_3 are increased. Metabolic alkalosis is caused by vomiting, excessive intake of antacids, and gastric suctioning. The symptoms are tingling, irritability, confusion, tetany, decreased respirations, and muscle cramping. Potassium is also decreased. **Nursing interventions are to**

administer IV fluids, monitor electrolytes, increase potassium, and treat the underlying cause.

Respiratory acidosis	Increase in $PaCO_2$ (>45 mmHg)	Decrease in pH (<7.35)
Respiratory alkalosis	Decrease in $PaCO_2$ (<35 mmHg)	Increase in pH (>7.45)
Metabolic acidosis	Decrease in pH (<7.35)	Decrease in HCO_3 (<22 mEq/L)
Metabolic alkalosis	Increase in pH (>7.35)	Increase in HCO_3 (>26 mEq/L)

Understanding acid–base imbalances was a challenge when I was taking this course. Study groups were definitely very helpful. Memorizing this chart will help you match the imbalance with the corresponding values. Online, you can find many acronyms for the imbalances—try to Google acid–base imbalances.

FLUIDS AND ELECTROLYTES

Hydration is the key to keeping the body fluid and electrolytes balanced. When electrolytes are imbalanced, symptoms such as tachycardia, muscle cramping, or arrhythmias may occur. Electrolytes include sodium, potassium, magnesium, calcium, and phosphorus. Memorize the lab values for electrolytes because you will need to know them for the rest of your nursing career. I know what you are thinking: "Oh, man, more things to remember." Yes, more things to remember. It seems like a lot now, but once you become familiar with the values, it will get easier. As a nurse, you will find there are little cheats on the computer that will give you the lab values, so it does get easier. In school, there are no little cheat sheets, so you must memorize! I will describe each electrolyte in detail for you step by step. Let's begin, shall we?

Electrolyte Lab Values:

- Potassium (K): 3.5–5.0 mEq/L
- Sodium (Na): 135–145 mEq/L
- Magnesium (Mg): 1.5–2.6 mg/dL
- Phosphorus (P): 2.7–4.5 mg/dL
- Calcium (Ca): 8.6–10.4 mg/dL

Here is a little secret: The most tested electrolytes are potassium and sodium. Remember all of the lab values, but concentrate and understand K and Na. In the following section, we describe the imbalances.

Fluid Imbalances

Dehydration/Hypovolemia

Dehydration or hypovolemia is a loss of fluid volume. Causes of dehydration are poor nutrition or fluid intake, surgery, diarrhea, renal disease, vomiting, NGT suctioning, and diuretics. Patients may present with symptoms of increased HR, decreased BP, poor skin turgor, weight loss, low urine output, dizziness, and weakness. Treatment for dehydration is to increase oral intake and to administer intravenous fluids. Monitor intake and urine output.

Fluid Overload/Hypervolemia

An excess of fluid is called hypervolemia. **Too much fluid can cause edema (swelling in the intravascular space), typically seen in the lower extremities and ankles, or crackles in the lungs.** Hypervolemia can be caused by renal disease or congestive heart failure. Symptoms include crackles in the lungs, edema (swelling in the body), bounding pulse, weight gain, increased BP, and shortness of breath. Treatment consists of administering a diuretic such as furosemide (Lasix), discontinuing all intravenous fluids, decreasing fluid intake, monitoring strict intake and output, monitoring daily weights, and cardiac monitoring.

Potassium Imbalances

Hypokalemia

In this condition, the potassium level is below 3.5 mEq/L. Hypokalemia can be caused by vomiting, diarrhea, gastric suctioning, kidney disease, and diuretics. Symptoms include irregular pulse, heart arrhythmias, muscle weakness, and muscle cramping. Treatment includes administering oral potassium, and intravenous fluids with potassium. Oral potassium is very bitter, so mix in a cup of orange juice to mask the taste. Cardiac monitoring is necessary. **Patients with hypokalemia usually have an EKG pattern with a depressed U wave. IV potassium is mixed with saline given only at a slow rate, over the course of two or more hours. Never push IV potassium, because it tends to burn and cause discomfort.** Monitor the patient's kidney status closely before administering potassium.

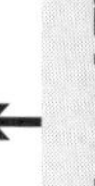

Hyperkalemia

Here, potassium levels are above 5.0 mEq/L. Hyperkalemia is caused by kidney disease, and medications such as angiotensin-converting enzyme (ACE) inhibitors are common causes. Symptoms include slow HR, weakness, cardiac arrhythmias, abdominal cramping, and muscle twitching. → **A peaked T wave may appear on the EKG**; this cardiac arrhythmia can be fatal and must be treated immediately. Treatment includes decreasing potassium in the diet and administering sodium polystyrene (Kayexalate), a medication that decreases potassium in the blood.

Sodium Imbalances

Hyponatremia

In this condition, sodium levels are below 135 mEq/L. Hyponatremia is caused by fluid overload, edema, diuretics, burns/wounds, and administration of an excess amount of D5W. Symptoms include headache, confusion, abdominal cramping, muscle cramps, nausea, dry mucous membranes, and clammy skin. Treatment consists of administering IV fluids with sodium. Medications such as tolvaptan (Samsca) may be administered to increase sodium. Monitor sodium levels.

Hypernatremia

Here, sodium levels are above 145 mEq/L. Hypernatremia is caused by dehydration and an increase in salt intake. Symptoms include edema, weight gain, thirst, weakness, and fatigue. Treatment consists of monitoring sodium intake, administering diuretics to remove sodium, and monitoring daily weights.

Magnesium Imbalances

Hypomagnesemia

In this condition, magnesium levels are below 1.5 mg/dL. An increase in Mg levels can be caused by alcoholism, vomiting, gastric suctioning, medications, and poor nutrition. Symptoms include increase in BP, positive Chvostek's and Trousseau's signs, mental status changes, and tremors. A positive Chvostek's sign is identified by muscle contraction in the face. When the facial nerve is tapped, usually in the jaw, there is a twitch on the nose or mouth. Trousseau's sign is identified by applying and inflating a BP cuff; a positive sign produces an abnormal spasm in the arm.

Treatment consists of increasing Mg levels by administering magnesium sulfate (high-alert medication) intravenously as ordered.

Hypermagnesemia

Here, magnesium levels are above 2.5 mg/dL. An increase in magnesium is caused by too much Mg in the diet, renal failure, or adrenal insufficiency. Symptoms include muscle weakness, decreased HR, respiratory depression, decreased reflexes, and GI upset. **Treatment consists of administering calcium gluconate intravenously. Monitor the patient's level of consciousness and monitor for confusion.** ←

Phosphorus Imbalances

Hypophosphatemia

In this condition, the phosphorus level is less than 2.7 mg/dL. Causes of decreased phosphorus are lack of nutrition, increased calcium levels, thyroid disorders, alcoholism, and poor nutrition. Symptoms include muscle weakness, respiratory depression, irritability, and positive Chvostek's and Trousseau's signs. Treatment consists of oral phosphorus with vitamin D as the first line of treatment.

Hyperphosphatemia

Here, phosphorus levels are above 4.5 mg/dL. Causes of increased phosphorus are renal disorders, thyroid disorders, and a **decrease in calcium levels that increases phosphorus**. Treatment consists of administering a calcium-containing phosphate binder such as Renagel and Phoslo. ←

Calcium Imbalances

Hypocalcemia

In this condition, calcium levels are below 8.6 mg/dL. Hypocalcemia is caused by thyroid disorders, renal failure, vitamin D deficiency, increased phosphorus, and chemotherapy. Symptoms are muscle numbness and tingling, positive Chvostek's and Trousseau's signs, seizures, and muscle twitching. Treatment consists of administering calcium and vitamin D.

Hypercalcemia

Here, calcium levels are above 10.4 mg/dL. Hypercalcemia is caused by overactive thyroid, cancer, and diuretics. Symptoms are muscle weakness, weight loss, confusion, nausea, kidney stones, and abdominal pain. Treatment consists of calcitonin, loop diuretics, and bisphosphonates such as etidronate.

INTRAVENOUS FLUIDS

Several different types of intravenous fluids are used to replace electrolyte imbalances:

Isotonic Solutions: Isotonic fluids are used to treat dehydration and metabolic acidosis. The types of isotonic fluids are 0.9% sodium chloride (the most commonly given fluid), lactated Ringer's solution, and 5% dextrose in water (D5W).

Hypotonic Solutions: Hypotonic solutions have low osmotic pressure and are used to treat edema and hypotension. Types of hypotonic solutions are 0.45% normal saline (NS) and 5% dextrose.

Hypertonic Solutions: Hypertonic solutions have high osmotic pressure and are used to treat blood loss, hypovolemia, and hyponatremia. They are usually given at a slow rate to decrease the risk of fluid overload. Types of hypertonic solutions are dextrose 5% in 0.45% NS, dextrose 5% in 0.9% NS, and dextrose 5% in lactated Ringer's.

When administering intravenous fluids (IVF), follow the physician's orders and administer the correct rate. IVF are given through an IV site, and it is important to assess the site for redness, infiltration, or swelling.

INTRAVENOUS SITES

Intravenous lines are started on patients for a number of reasons. They allow health care professionals to administer medications, procedures, surgery, and fluids. Most hospital protocols require all patients to have IV access. An IV is best started in the distal veins of the arms and needs to be large enough to maintain the catheter. A 22-gauge needle is most commonly used. A 20-gauge needle is used for patients receiving blood products or requiring contrast. IV sites must be changed every 2 to 3 days. Complications of IVs include infiltration (swelling of the site due to fluid in the tissues) and phlebitis (inflammation of the vein). It is the nurse's responsibility to assess the IV site and change the site if any problems occur.

→ **Peripherally inserted central catheter (PICC) lines** are used for patients who are on long-term antibiotics or if intravenous sites cannot be obtained. A PICC line is inserted through the cephalic or brachial vein and then advanced into the superior vena cava. A chest x-ray is used to confirm placement. A PICC line dressing must be changed every 7 days. Arm circumference is measured daily. If swelling or edema occurs in the arm, an ultrasound may be needed to see whether blood exists in the arm. Blood draws are allowed in PICC lines.

A subclavian Port-a-Cath is a central venous catheter that goes into the vein in the chest wall and into the heart. Dressing on the port is changed every 7 days. Aseptic technique is needed when changing and accessing the port. Blood draws are also allowed. Port-a-Cath use is common with patients receiving chemotherapy or frequent transfusions. ←

MEDICATION ADMINISTRATION

Nursing has three main tasks. The first is to assess the patient, the second is to administer medications ordered by the physician, and the third is documentation. It is important to know the five rights of medication administration and carefully administer medications as ordered. The five rights of medication administration are right patient, right drug, right route, right dose, and right time. Using the five rights ensures the patient's safety and prevents you from administering the wrong medication.

Pharmacology is one of the hardest courses in nursing school, but one of the most important. You will need the information you learn in this class for the rest of your nursing career. I know you are probably staring at your notes and textbook, saying, "How on earth am I going to remember all of this?" It is possible. There are tons of tips and helpful secrets in Chapter 5 that will help. Medications are typically given orally, intravenously, intramuscularly, or subcutaneously. Be careful with patients who are at risk for aspiration or have difficulty swallowing; these patients may require medications to be crushed or given intravenously. Always assess, describe, and make sure the patient is aware of the medications you are administering. When administering cardiac medications, always obtain a BP/pulse and follow parameters.

During this course, I was a nervous wreck. The thought of giving a patient a shot would make me so nervous. I think it is because I am not too fond of shots myself that I felt awful giving them to my patients. My hands would shake, and I would start sweating and begin having a mini anxiety attack when my instructor would say it was time to start an IV or give a subcutaneous shot. But I am here to tell you that you will overcome this fear! Once you begin to gain confidence and practice, you will become a pro in no time. The first time I gave a subcutaneous heparin shot, my hands were shaky, and I seemed like a mess inside while trying to stay calm on the outside. By the end of the course, I no longer felt nervous and gained enough confidence to comfortably administer shots. All it takes is a little practice and positive self-talk.

INFECTION CONTROL AND PREVENTION

Infections are invasions of organisms such as viruses, bacteria, and parasites that enter the body. In all health care facilities, aseptic techniques are used to prevent the transmission of these organisms. Standard precautions consist of hand washing and the use of gloves when in contact with patients. There are different types of precautions based on the type of infection.

Standard Precautions: Standard precautions are used for all contact with patients. Wash hands and use gloves with all patients.

Contact Precautions: Contact precautions are the use of gown and gloves. Methicillin-resistant *Staphylococcus aureus* (MRSA), *Clostridium difficile* (*C. diff*), shingles, vancomycin resistant enterococci (VRE), and *E. coli* in the urine are common infections that require contact precautions. When treating patients with *C-diff*, you must wash your hands with soap and water to prevent infection; hand sanitizer does not kill the *C-diff* bacteria. Pregnant women or caregivers who have not had or been vaccinated against chickenpox (varicella) should not care for patients with shingles. Always throw gowns away before exiting the room, and wash your hands thoroughly.

Droplet Precautions: These require the use of gown, gloves, eye shield (if preferred), and mask. An N95 mask is needed and fitted by size. Patients who have TB or Ebola require droplet precautions. A negative pressure room is also needed. Droplets are found in secretions such as cough or other bodily fluids.

Airborne Precautions: These require the use of gown, gloves, and mask. A regular surgical mask can be worn. Patients who test positive for influenza require airborne precautions.

There are many pathogens, viruses, and infectious diseases that require precautions. I have listed the most common types above. Please refer to your textbook and class notes for further details and information. Remember it is important to wash hands and use standard precautions with all patients. Keep yourself safe!

THE SURGICAL EXPERIENCE

There are three main phases of the surgical experience: (a) preoperative, (b) intraoperative, and (c) postoperative. In the following section, I describe each phase in detail, highlighting the most important information. With each phase, aseptic and sterile techniques are used. Hand washing is very important! Hand washing is used on the unit and through all phases of the surgical experience.

Preoperative Phase

The preoperative phase begins with the decision to consent to surgery and ends when the patient is transferred into the operating room. Before any procedure, it is important to have the patient sign consent for surgery, and to ensure that all lab work has been completed, vital signs are stable, and the patient understands the surgical procedure. The nurse's role in preparation for the day of surgery is to make sure all the consents are signed, prep the patient for surgery, assess vital signs and labs, remove jewelry, prepare the bowel/bladder (making sure the patient voids before going to surgery), ensure all preoperative medications are given, and make sure all the patient's questions are answered. **It is very important to administer BP medications and antibiotics prior to surgery. Beta blockers must be given if it is within parameters. If the BP is low, the surgeon should be contacted.** ←

Patient education is important, and the patient must be taught what to expect preoperatively, intraoperatively, and postoperatively. Preoperatively, you need to discuss the procedure and educate the patient on ways to avoid complications postoperatively. **Some of the main points that need to be addressed with patients to prepare them for the postop phase are to turn and reposition in bed every 2 hours in order to increase circulation, and to apply SCDs and TEDs in order to decrease the risk of blood clots. Encourage the patient to cough and deep breathe, and consider using an incentive spirometer to increase lung expansion and decrease the chances of developing hospital-acquired pneumonia.** ← Preventing complications is vital, and educating patients is important for a speedy recovery.

Intraoperative Phase

This phase begins with the patient being transferred from preop to the operating room and ends in the postanesthesia care unit (PACU). In this phase, the surgeon performs the procedure. Nurses play many roles in the intraoperative phase. In the operating room, there is a scrub nurse and a circulating nurse to help assist the surgeon with any needs. They help with handing and counting all the instruments and materials used. They also help monitor the patient during the surgical procedure. The intraoperative phase ends when the surgical procedure is completed.

Postoperative Phase

The postoperative stage begins when the patient arrives in the PACU and ends when the patient is placed in a medical–surgical unit. The postoperative phase is a critical phase where the nurse must monitor for any postop complications or any acute changes. The PACU nurse is responsible for maintaining the patient's airway, assessing the wound or incision, controlling pain, monitoring urinary output, assessing vital signs, and assessing for any changes in the patient's mental status. It is the nurse's responsibility to convey any changes to the surgeon immediately.

→ **The most common postsurgical complications are shock, hemorrhage, pneumonia, wound infections, and blood clots.** In the preoperative phase, postop teaching was completed, with the goal of helping the patient understand these complications and learn how to decrease the chances of complications by using the numerous preventive measures. Once the patient arrives on a medical–surgical unit, it is the floor nurse's responsibility to continue to assess for postop complications and any changes that might occur.

BLOOD TRANSFUSIONS

Blood transfusions are needed for the patient with a decrease in hemoglobin and hematocrit. Conditions such as sickle cell disease, cancer, GI bleeds, and anemia can all cause a decrease in these levels. Blood transfusion is administered to increase these levels. A consent form must first be signed, there must be a physician's order, and all complications must be explained. A cross-match is needed. The blood is prepared and refrigerated until transfusion. An IV site is needed. Two nurses are needed to check the blood. Obtain vital signs before the transfusion,

15 minutes into the transfusion, and after the transfusion. If the patient has an abnormal temperature, Tylenol may be given before the transfusion. Assess for a reaction to the blood. Sit in the room for 15 minutes once the transfusion has started. If a reaction occurs, call the physician immediately and stop the blood.

SEE YOU LATER FUNDAMENTALS!

Congrats! You have completed the first course in nursing! You deserve a pat on the back, and more. This was a tough course to get through, and there is so much to learn, but learning is what nursing is all about. I hope this chapter has helped you to highlight all the important information. Pay attention to what your professors recommend as important content to study and learn. They are the ones who make the exams, so pay close attention! Try not to miss too many classes; professors love to drop little hints in class as to what might be on the exam. Remember, this is a tiny study guide with a big punch, but each course is designed differently; use this book as a guideline along with your class notes and textbook.

In fundamentals of nursing, you will also be attending your first clinical. You will apply all this information in a hospital or nursing home setting. The sections not reviewed in this book that you will need to know are how to wash your hands thoroughly and make a patient's bed. You will also be getting your first pair of scrubs. Now, I may sound like a nerd, but I was so excited to finally wear scrubs and attend a clinical, almost like I was in *Grey's Anatomy* or something. It feels good when you study so hard and finally get to use all this knowledge to begin your nursing career. Just a little side note: If you are having difficulty or need a little extra help, talk to your professor—this would be the best time. Study sessions are a great help. (Also, some students at this point figure out that this might not be the right field for them—if this is the case for you, speak to your counselor, and don't worry, because there are always other options.)

You should be proud: You have completed the first course, and you are on your way to becoming a great nurse. Let's bring on health assessment!

TWO

HEALTH ASSESSMENT

Health assessment is by far one of the best courses in nursing school. There are few or no exams in this class—rather, it is hands on, and at the end of the course, you are able to complete a full head-to-toe assessment on a patient for your final grade. This class goes right along with the anatomy and physiology course, but in a way that is a little less textbook-based and more hands on. This course will teach you how to perform a detailed assessment on each part of the adult body. (Pediatric health assessment will be discussed in Chapter 6.) You will be able to identify any abnormalities, how to document your assessment, and understand how a full-body assessment is performed. The exams or tests in this course are a little different. Each week you will learn an assessment on one or more parts of the body. At the end of each week, you will have to perform your assessment for a test grade. At the end of the course, the final exam is how well you perform physical assessment, including identifying any problems that could occur during the assessment.

Remember that each course is designed differently, and keep notes on what your professor highlights. The best part about this course is that you can practice on friends, family, and pretty much anyone who allows you to do so. If you are having difficulties during this course, practice your assessment techniques when you have time, and attend study sessions, if possible. You will use the information in this class throughout your nursing career. The most important part of our job is the assessment. It is important to assess, document, and notify the doctor of any changes that occur. For example, you may notice swelling in a patient's bilateral extremity. This information is based on your physical assessment of the patient. Nurses are usually the first to recognize changes in a patient's condition, and a detailed exam is very important during the shift. At the beginning of each assessment, it is important to explain to the patient what you are doing and provide privacy while performing the assessment. If a patient is admitted with a respiratory complication or abdominal pain, you need to focus more closely on those areas during your assessment.

→ **This whole section is going to be highlighted. Each section of this course is tested information. A complete physical assessment will be your final exam.** Good luck and enjoy. Take out those stethoscopes and flashlights; it's time to assess.

SKIN, HAIR, AND NAILS

The skin is the largest organ in the body and acts as a barrier against many pathogens. Think of the skin as a protective shield. → **The structure of the skin is divided into three layers: (a) epidermis, (b) dermis, and (c) subcutaneous layer**. Details of the layers of the skin will not be tested or focused on. If you refer back to your anatomy and physiology textbook, you can get a better understanding of each layer and the role they play in the body. Let's continue with the assessment of the skin.

Skin Assessment

First, start the assessment by providing privacy for the patient—shut doors or close curtains to provide privacy. Explain that you will be performing a physical assessment on the whole body. Use standard precautions when assessing any patient. Ask the patient to lie down on the bed, and begin assessing the skin on each section of the body. Assess the skin by looking at the color, texture, temperature, and any abnormalities. → **Skin turgor—that is, elasticity of the skin—is assessed. If, upon being gently pinched, the skin (usually on the hand) does not retract to its normal state or takes slightly longer, this can be a sign of dehydration**. Skin that is assessed with no abnormalities is documented as dry and intact, meaning it is normal. Obtain a little history from the patient about their skin before your assessment. The common skin abnormalities are listed below; refer to your textbook for pictures to gain a better understanding.

- Ecchymosis: This is bruising of the skin. It appears black and blue and is typically seen on the upper extremities. It is commonly seen in elderly patients as well as in patients who have fragile skin.
- → **Jaundice: This is a yellow-tinged color of the skin that is caused by liver failure or liver disease.**
- Erythema: This is redness to an affected area caused by cellulitis (common skin infection), skin infection, rash, or irritation of the skin. The area of redness can be large or small.
- Pruritus: This is a rash that is itchy and typically patchy; it is caused by an allergic reaction.

- **Cyanosis: This is a blue-tinged color that is typically seen at the tips of fingers or toes; it is caused by a lack of oxygen and blood flow.** ←
- Skin tears: An opening of the top layer of the skin causing a break in the skin. Usually seen in patients with fragile skin or in patients who are on the medication prednisone, which causes paper-thin skin.
- Ulcers/wounds: Opening of the skin that is identified by stages. Refer to Chapter 1 or 3 for more details. These wounds are commonly found in the elderly population or immobile patients.
- Abrasion/laceration: An abrasion is superficial damage to the skin, such as a scrape.
- Skin lesions: There are many forms of lesions that can appear on the skin:
  - A *macule* is a flat lesion that is less than 1 cm
  - A *papule* is a raised firm lesion less than 1 cm
  - A *plaque* is an elevated lesion that is greater than 1 cm
  - A *nodule* is a firm lesion greater than 1 cm
  - A *vesicle* is an elevated capsule that contains straw-colored fluid and is greater than 1 cm.
  - A *bulla* is a fluid-filled lesion that measures less than 1 cm and resembles a blister.

When documenting skin findings, it is important to describe where any abnormality was found, the size, color, odor, and if there is any drainage. Take pictures of all wounds and record exact measurements. Normal skin findings are documented as dry and intact. An example of an abnormal finding is left upper arm ecchymosis, a skin lesion on right arm, or a dime-size erythema on calf. Report all findings to your instructor.

Hair Assessment

Begin with assessing the scalp—inspect the scalp by running your fingers through it and palpating for any changes. The hair should be full and clean. Common hair disorders are alopecia, which is hair loss (other than normal, age-appropriate hair loss) and can be caused by chemotherapy; or dry coarse hair, which can signify a thyroid problem. Assess the scalp for any cuts or abrasions. Document the findings.

Nail Assessment

Nails are usually a great indicator of respiratory or circulatory problems. A lack of blood flow or venous insufficiency can be determined by nail color. Assess the patient's nail color. Remove any nail polish. Nails should be clean and normal in color, and capillary refill should be less than 3 seconds. The capillary refill test is a quick way to see if there is proper blood flow to the fingers. It is done by pressing down on the nail. When pressure is applied, the nails turns white, and the nail should return to pink in less than 3 seconds. If not, this could be a sign of dehydration or a vascular problem.

Nail abnormalities include:

- Clubbing: Ridges in the nails can signify a decrease in oxygen.
- Cyanosis: A blue tinge to the nails can also mean there is a decrease in oxygen and blood flow to the nail bed.
- Spooning: A curve in the nail can be a sign of a lack of nutrients or iron.
- White bands: White bands that are seen on the nails can be caused by cirrhosis of the liver or liver disorders.

Document all your findings!

HEAD, EARS, AND NOSE

Start the assessment by palpating the facial bones and skull for any abnormalities, lesions, or pain. If possible, have the patient sit on the edge of the bed to assess the back of the head as well. Stand in front of the patient and assess for symmetry of the nose, eyes, ears, and mouth. A deviation or drooping can be a sign of a stroke or other neurological disorder. Obtain a history from the patient before documenting any abnormalities. A facial droop may be a result of a past stroke. Cranial nerves will come into play during this section and many more. (Pay attention: I have highlighted them in the chapter for you.)

Eye Assessment

First, obtain a history from the patient of any eye disorders. Ask the patient if he or she wears glasses or contact lenses or has any history of blindness. Assess the eye for visual acuity, symmetry, lids, lashes, sclera, cornea, and pupil response, and palpate around the eye for any pain. Assess the eye for redness and drainage. The eye has many different assessment points that we will discuss.

- Visual acuity (cranial nerve II) determines how well the patient is able to see. This is measured using the Snellen chart and by asking the patient to cover one eye while reading the chart from a distance. Normal vision is 20/20. Patients may already wear glasses and be aware that they have difficulty seeing.

- Assess the sclera, the white part of the eye. The iris is the colored portion of the eye. **Jaundice is seen in the sclera and is a common finding in patients with liver disorders.**
- Assess the palpebral fissure, which is the eyelid. Abnormality such as ptosis (droopy eye) may be seen. Exophthalmos is bulging of the eyes, seen in patients who suffer from Graves' disease, a thyroid disorder.
- Inspect the conjunctiva by pulling the upper and lower lids, looking for complications such as conjunctivitis or hemorrhage.
- **Assess the pupil size, shape, and equality (cranial nerve III). The size of the pupil can vary between 2 and 4 mm.**
- Assess for extraocular movements (cranial nerves III, IV, and VI) by creating a letter "H" with the penlight, and having the patient follow the shape to show the pupils' ability to follow the configuration. A lack of coordination to follow the "H" can indicate disorders such as nystagmus and strabismus (lazy eye).

Assessment of the Pupils

- Direct assessment: Instruct the patient to look straight ahead, and shine a light directly into each pupil starting from the temporal side (from the forehead down to the pupil). In response to the light, the pupils should constrict quickly, meaning go from large to small; this is the pupil's reaction to adjusting to the light. A fixed or dilated pupil means the pupils remain the same size and do not constrict in response to the light. The term for this is *pinpoint*. This can signify neurological damage, head injury, intoxication, or a reaction to medications.
- Consensual assessment: Instruct the patient to look straight ahead. Shine a light starting from the temporal side, and assess for constriction of the opposite eye. When one pupil is stimulated by light, the opposite pupil also constricts.
- Near reaction assessment: Instruct the patient to look straight ahead. Shine a light into each eye, and look for dilation and constriction of both pupils.

Document your findings and report any abnormalities during your assessment.

Ear Assessment

Obtain a history of any ear disorders or problems from the patient. Ask the patient whether he or she is hard of hearing. Assess hearing, external ear, and internal ear, and palpate the outer ear for any abnormalities.

→ • **Inspect the ear by gently pulling the pinna back and up.** The pinna is the top of the ear where it begins to curve; refer to your textbook for a visual.
- Use an otoscope to assess inside the ear, looking for any abnormalities such as swelling or drainage. Identify the tympanic membrane (a pearly gray structure in the ear). Inspect the external ear for any lesions or tenderness.
- Conduct the hearing test known as the *whisper test* (cranial nerve VIII). Instruct the patient to cover one ear while you stand about 1 to 2 feet away. Whisper two words or numbers in the uncovered ear while asking the patient to repeat the word or number back. Conduct the test on both sides.
- Document any findings and report any abnormalities.

Nose Assessment

Obtain a history of any nasal disorders or problems.

- Inspect the interior and exterior of the nose. The nose should appear symmetrical, patent, and nondeviated.
- Palpate the sinuses by gently pressing on the frontal and maxillary sinuses, assessing for any tenderness or pain. Patients with sinus infection often feel tenderness and pressure.
- Assess for any bleeding or injury to the nose. Document the findings.

MOUTH AND LIPS

Obtain a history of any mouth or lip disorders. Inspect the lips, making sure there are no abnormalities. The lips should appear moist with no lesions or cracks.

- Inspect the teeth and gums. The gums should appear moist and pink in color. They should have no lesions. The teeth should be intact with no cracks; assess for toothaches.
- Dry mucous membranes, cracked lips, and dry mouth can be signs of dehydration.

- Assess the uvula (the soft tissue that hangs at the back of the throat). Make sure the uvula is midline and rises when swallowing.
- Have the patient smile, making sure there is no deviation; a droop can signify a stroke or cerebrovascular accident (CVA).
- Document the findings.

NECK AND NODES ASSESSMENT

First obtain a history of any neck abnormalities.

- Assess the neck, and palpate for any lesions and enlarged nodes. The trachea should appear midline.
- Assess the carotid arteries one at a time. Never assess both carotids together as it can cause severe dizziness.
- Palpate the thyroid gland. Enlarged thyroids may be signs of hyperthyroidism, goiter, or other abnormalities. Enlarged nodes need to be assessed and reported to the physician.
- Document the findings.

NEUROLOGICAL SYSTEM AND CRANIAL NERVES

Obtain a history (pretty repetitive, I know). The neurological system is very complex and coordinates many functions in the body. This section will cover the five main tests used to perform an accurate neurological exam: (a) level of consciousness (LOC), (b) cranial nerves, (c) motor function, (d) sensory function, and (e) deep tendon reflexes.

Level of Consciousness

Assess the patient's mental status. Ask the patient to identify self, place, and time. If there is no alteration in mental status, document the findings as "patient is alert and oriented times 3." If the patient is slightly confused and cannot state the time or place, document the findings as "patient is alert and oriented times 2 or 1," meaning they are slightly confused. Older patients with dementia (e.g., Alzheimer's) often show declines in mental status and the ability to answer questions appropriately. Assess for any new changes in mental status, slurred speech (sign of stroke), and, in older patients, urinary tract infections (UTI), which can alter a patient's mental status. It is always important to obtain labs and urine cultures.

Cranial Nerves

So sorry to break it to you, but you will be tested on the 12 cranial nerves! Cranial nerves originate from the brain and perform different functions in the body. The cranial nerves are:

- Cranial nerve I: The *olfactory* nerve functions in the sense of smell.
- Cranial nerve II: The *optic* nerve functions in the ability to see. Visual acuity and visual fields are assessed.
- Cranial nerve III: The *oculomotor* nerve functions in pupil response and lid movement. Assess by the response of the eyes to light.
- Cranial nerve IV: The *trochlear* nerve functions in eye movement. It is assessed by testing extraocular movements using the cardinal fields of gaze.
- Cranial nerve V: The *trigeminal sensory* nerve is the largest cranial nerve and plays a role in the sensory function of the nose, eyes, tongue, and teeth. This is assessed by applying a light touch to the cheek, forehead, and jaw. Typically, the end of a cotton swab is used on the three dermatomes, while asking the patient if he or she is able to feel the sensation. The patient should also be asked to clench the jaw, to assess for muscle strength.
- Cranial nerve VI: The *abducens* nerve performs the function of the lateral eye movement. It is assessed by using the cardinal field of gaze.
- Cranial nerve VII: The *facial motor* nerve functions in the ability to perform facial expressions. It is assessed by having the patient smile, clench teeth, and wrinkle the forehead.
- Cranial nerve VIII: The *acoustic* nerve functions in the ability to hear. Assess the patient's ability to hear by using the whisper test. This can determine whether the patient is hard of hearing.
- Cranial nerve IX/X: The *glossopharyngeal/vagus* nerve controls the tongue and palate. Assess the patient's ability to swallow produce the gag reflex.
- Cranial nerve XI: The *spinal accessory* nerve governs head control. Assess by having the patient turn his or her head and pressing against the shoulders, assessing for resistance and strength.
- Cranial nerve X: The *hypoglossal* nerve controls the tongue function. Assess by having the patient stick his or her tongue out and making sure the tongue is midline.

Document any findings.

Motor Function

Motor function is the ability to evaluate the strength of muscles in the upper and lower extremities. To examine the upper extremities, ask the patient to press against your arms while assessing the strength of each arm. Strength should be equal in both arms. To assess the lower extremities, ask the patient to press his or her legs against your hands, assessing for strength and resistance. Strength should be equal in both legs.

To assess whether the patient has a steady or unsteady gait, ask the patient to walk in a straight line. While the patient is walking, assess for weakness or the inability to ambulate. Document any findings.

Sensory Function

Sensory function is the body's response to light touch, vibration, and pain sensations. *Light touch* is assessed by using a cotton ball to touch the major dermatomes while looking at the response to the sensation. *Vibration* is assessed by using a tuning fork to apply sensation, and asking the patient if he or she can feel the vibration. To elicit the sensations of pain, gently use a paper clip or the end of a tongue blade.

Document the findings.

Deep Tendon Reflexes

Deep tendon reflexes are the response of reflexes in the triceps, biceps, brachioradialis, patellar, and Achilles tendon. This response is assessed by gently tapping on the reflex to stimulate a response. The response of reflexes is graded as follows: 4+ indicates a brisk and hyperactive response, 2+ is a normal response, and 0 means no response. Document the findings.

THORAX AND LUNGS

The thorax and lungs are a little difficult to describe in writing; they are best visualized, but I will try my best. First obtain a health history of any respiratory disorders the patient may have. Pay close attention to the instructor's assessment of the thorax and lungs. Assess the lungs and thorax, noting any abnormalities.

- Begin the assessment by positioning the patient upright or asking the patient to sit up. Before auscultating lung sounds, turn off the television and shut the room door. The fewer distractions, the better. Time to get those stethoscopes!

I will describe the lung assessment in four steps for easy learning.

- The first step is to assess the lungs, looking for symmetry, use of accessory muscles (apparent when the patient is experiencing distress), and diameter of the lungs. Assess to make sure the patient is not having difficulty breathing or in distress. Common conditions that can alter the lungs' diameter are kyphosis, chronic obstructive pulmonary disease (COPD), and emphysema, to name just a few.
- Second, palpate the chest wall by placing your hands on the posterior chest, and assess vibrations, which should be equal throughout.
- Third, percuss the chest wall by gently tapping on the chest. Normal sounds are loud and hollow. If there is air or fluid in the lungs, it will sound dull and filled. Dull percussions can mean there is a pleural effusion or fluid overload in the lungs.
- The fourth step is the auscultation of the lung sounds. Get those stethoscopes out! **Always auscultate lung sounds on the patient's bare skin—never auscultate over clothing.** When listening to breath sounds, you are to listen to the lower lungs and upper lungs on each side, that is, the right and left, equaling four sections on the lung field. Place the stethoscopes on the chest, making sure the room is quiet, and listen carefully. Have the patient take a deep breath for each region. You should hear air moving through the lung clearly; this is normal. Abnormal breath sounds are crackles, ronchi, wheezing, rales, diminished, or rubbing. These breath sounds can mean numerous conditions. Ronchi or coarse breath sounds can be due to pneumonia or upper respiratory infection. Crackles can signify fluid in the lungs. Wheezing can signify asthma. Report any of these findings to your instructor. Document your findings.

HEART AND PERIPHERAL VASCULAR ASSESSMENT

Cardiac Assessment

Obtain a history from the patient, asking the patient if he or she has had any cardiovascular disorders, arrhythmias, or other problems. The heart assessment goes right along with listening to the lungs. While listening to the lungs, you need to listen to the heart at the same time. There are four areas where heartbeats can be heard:

- Aortic area: Right second intercostal at the sternal border.
- Pulmonic area: Left second intercostal; this is where S1 and S2 are strongly heard.

- Tricuspid area: Left third to fourth intercostal.
- Mitral area: Left fifth intercostal space at the midclavicular line.

When listening to these regions, the heart sounds should be strong and 60 to 100 bpm. Abnormal lung sounds are murmurs or arrhythmias, which may be new or chronic for the patient. The most commonly heard arrhythmia is atrial fibrillation, which causes an irregular heartbeat.

The Peripheral Vascular Assessment

The peripheral vascular system consists of all arteries and veins in the body that circulate blood, specifically, in the upper and lower extremities. I will describe to you the various pulses to assess, but a visual picture will be needed for a better understanding. The pulses are brachial, radial, femoral, popliteal, posterior tibial, and dorsalis pedis. There are many conditions where pulses are either hard to palpate or weak, such as vascular disease or edema. A Doppler stethoscope is then used to feel and hear the pulse. The most common pulse assessed in adults and infants is the brachial.

Document your findings!

MUSCULOSKELETAL ASSESSMENT

Obtain a health history from the patient, assessing for any musculoskeletal disorders or injuries. The musculoskeletal assessment is a head-to-toe assessment; it is helpful to perform the assessment in this order so you will not forget anything when tested. So, let's start with the head.

- Inspect the head for symmetry, deformities, bruising, or swelling. Palpate the head, assessing for warmth, tenderness, or pain. Ask the patient to move the head while assessing the neck for any abnormalities.
- Assess the temporomandibular joint (at the jaw). Inspect this joint by first locating the mandible and temporal bone. Inspect for symmetry. Palpate the joint while the patient moves and relaxes the jaw. Ask the patient to move his or her jaw from side to side, assessing for any deviations or pain in the jaw. A common disorder is lockjaw.
- Next assess the cervical spine and anterior neck. With the patient standing, ask him or her to tilt the head forward and backward. Assess the neck for symmetry, pain, muscle spasms, or tenderness. Then have the patient bend down and touch the knees, while you assess the curvature of the spine.

- Have the patient sit upright or at the edge of the bed. Assess the shoulders for symmetry and alignment. Run your hands along the shoulders, assessing for pain or discomfort. Next, assess range of motion (ROM) of the shoulders by having the patient stand up straight while asking him or her to flex, extend, abduct, and adduct the arms. Assess for any abnormalities.
- After inspecting the shoulders, move down to the elbows and wrist. Know the major bones in the arm such as the humerus and ulna. Inspect the elbow for swelling, pain, bruising, and any deformities. Similar to the shoulder, perform ROM of the arm, and assess for pain or limitations.
- The hand anatomy consists of several small bones, including those of the wrist and fingers. Assess the hand, and palpate each finger, assessing for any pain, swelling, or tenderness. A common complication such as rheumatoid arthritis can cause deformity and severe swelling in the hands and fingers.
- For the hip assessment, the patient will need to lie down. Perform ROM by having the patient move slightly from side to side, assessing for any pain, tenderness, and symmetry.
- The knee exam is pretty simple. Inspect the knee for any swelling, bruising, tenderness, or deformities. Evaluate ROM by extending the knee and then flexing to a 90° angle. Assess for any complications.
- Don't forget the ankles! They are the most overlooked during the assessment. Inspect the ankle for any deformities, swelling, or tenderness. Ask the patient to perform plantar flexion, dorsiflexion, inversion, and eversion of the ankle and foot, assessing for any abnormalities.
- Last but not least, assess the feet. Palpate the toes, assessing for any swelling, pain, or tenderness. Also note whether there are any calluses or bunions. If the patient is a diabetic, inspect the foot, carefully assessing for any cuts or ulcers. Diabetic patients often suffer from neuropathy of the feet (numbness), and are unable to feel if there is a cut or ulcer on the foot.
- Make sure to document and tell your instructor of any findings!

BREAST ASSESSMENT

Obtain a health history, paying attention to any surgeries such as breast implantation or mastectomy from breast cancer. Provide privacy for the patient while performing the assessment.

- First, assess the breast for symmetry. Assess the nipples for any discharge or fissures.

- Next, have the patient raise his or her arms; assess for symmetry, pain, or swelling.
- Palpate the breast, paying close attention to palpate for any lesions or lumps. Have the patient lie down and place his or her hands behind the head. Starting at the areola, gently compress the breast in a circle until your reach the armpit, assessing for any lumps or lesions. Next, assess the nipples for any discharge or pain.
- Breast exams are performed on both men and women. Men can also have masses and tenderness of the breast as well.

ABDOMINAL ASSESSMENT

Congratulations! You have made it to the last section of the health assessment.

Obtain a history from the patient. Ask the patient if he or she is having regular bowel movements, urinating frequently, and assess for pain in the abdomen. The abdomen is assessed in four quadrants:

- *Right upper quadrant* consists of the liver, gallbladder, and right kidney.
- *Right lower quadrant* consists of the colon, cecum, appendix, right ureter, and right spermatic cord.
- *Left upper quadrant* consists of the spleen, pancreas , and left kidney.
- *Left lower quadrant* consists of the sigmoid colon.

It is important to become familiar with the four quadrants so you know which structures you are assessing and palpating. Now, on to the assessment.

- First, inspect the outer abdomen and assess for distension. Distension of the abdomen can signify constipation, bowel obstruction, ileus, or pancreatitis. Auscultate each quadrant of the abdomen listening for bowel sounds, which sound like gurgling. Bowel sounds can be hyperactive, hypoactive, or normal. It is important that you hear bowel sounds in each quadrant. Bowel sounds signify that the stomach is digesting and motility is intact.
- After auscultation, percuss the abdomen. Place your hand palm down over the quadrants, and lightly tap your finger against your hand to make a tapping sound. Percuss each quadrant, listening for tympany, which is normal. Dullness is abnormal, and can signify a mass.

- The last step is palpation of the abdomen. Lightly press against each quadrant, assessing for pain or tenderness. Your instructor will also show you how to palpate and assess the liver. Document any findings.

We have completed the health assessment section. Congratulations! I know this chapter has tons of information, but it will all come together and make more sense as you perform the assessment either on your classmates or on patients during clinical. With practice, you will be able to identify abnormalities and perform a whole body assessment in a matter of minutes. I promise it will get easier.

As you have noticed, I did not highlight much content in this chapter because you are to become familiar with each section in order to perform a detailed assessment. The course is designed to go through one or more sections a week. The final exam is to perform a complete assessment for your instructor. A helpful tip is to start with the head and finish with the feet. Make notecards, and draw out the outline of the body and write down each assessment.

I was a nervous wreck during my assessments. I was always missing or skipping a part of the assessment. But the professors will prompt you at times to go over the missed section. So try to relax and stay calm—the more nervous you are, the easier it is to forget. Practice is key; spend some extra time in the lab going over the assessment with a friend. This was my favorite course in nursing school, and it is one of the most important. A nurse's main role is to assess and continue to look for any abnormalities that the patient may be experiencing and report any changes to the doctor. You will do great!

MEDICAL–SURGICAL NURSING

Oh, med–surg! Fancy meeting you here! Let's just say this is the most important course you will be taking in nursing school. I will not sugarcoat anything: It is also the most difficult, with tons of information packed into a semester. The PowerPoint slides are miles long (okay, this is a little bit of an exaggeration, but it seemed like it). Medical–surgical nursing goes over most conditions and disorders that can occur in the body, including definition, symptoms, diagnostics, complications, drug therapy, and nursing care. I know you might hear from other students about the difficulty of the course, but put those negative thoughts behind you. You need to begin the course with a positive attitude; you are smart and can pass this class. It will take some work on your part, though; organization and studying are the two main components needed to pass this class. Here are a few tips to help you with this class:

- Review the syllabus for the course. To be a step ahead, start reviewing the chapters. The med–surg book is huge! You will get an arm workout just from lugging this book around.
- Review the materials before class, and become familiar with the material you will need to know for that week. You do not want to be that student who has the face of a deer in the headlights; it isn't a cute look.
- Listen in class! Even though you may have had a late night prior to your 8 a.m. class or you just don't feel like being in class, try to pay attention. The professors often hint at what to expect on exams. This also means no texting or chatting, because you might miss something. I was not one to pay very close attention, and I was easily distracted in class. But, looking back, I wish I had paid closer attention; I think it would have helped me to know better what to expect on the exams. So, don't follow in my footsteps. Pay close attention.
- Do not study for the exams or quizzes the night before. The syllabus is there to let you know what to expect on exams and quizzes. Take your time in reviewing the material. You will

need this information forever, as a nursing student and as a nurse. Also, remember the ABCs (airway, breathing, and circulation). If your exams include any questions for which airway or breathing may be the answer, always choose this answer. → **When answering prioritization questions (which patient to help first) always choose the answer that pertains to the patient who is experiencing respiratory distress or whose airway is compromised.**

- Plan your partying and social events for weeks when your workload is not too great. Never plan social events for the night before an exam. These exams are usually count for 20% to 25% of your grade and are very hard to recover from if you do poorly on just one. Party and celebrate after you pass!

Use this study guide along with your class notes and textbook. I will highlight the most frequently tested conditions and disorders. Use your syllabus as a study guide. You can create note cards based on the different sections of the syllabus. I know this class can be overwhelming, but take it one step at a time. At most schools, tutors and study groups are available if you need a little extra help. Attending study groups shows the instructors you are trying, and usually extra credit is given. The material learned in this class prepares you for the clinical portion of this course as well.

Your class grade is based on two components: exams and how well you apply the information in clinical. The *class* is knowledge based, where you learn to use critical thinking skills. The *clinical* portion is where you apply your skills and perform nursing care. The clinical portion will give you a better understanding of what nurses really do: the assessment, administering medication, and documentation. You may grasp the concepts a little more easily when you perform them hands on and see the disorders and conditions up close. It is really exciting and makes you feel, "Yes, finally, this is what nursing is all about." Now take a deep breath: We are about to enter the world of med–surg. Hello, lab values.

IMPORTANT LAB VALUES

Lab values are used to help diagnose or help figure out what is going on with the patient by identifying key constiuents from a sample of either blood or urine. Sometimes a patient's problem cannot be physically assessed (i.e., through examination techniques or visual observation). In these cases, both blood work and urine testing can help diagnose a condition or problem the patient may be having. I wanted to start with lab values because they are mentioned very frequently throughout this chapter and are used as a diagnostic aid for each condition. Here are the normal lab values for an adult:

Lab Values:

Red blood cell (RBC) count: 4.5 to 6.0 $mm^3/\mu L$ in men/4.0 to 5.0 $mm^3/\mu L$ in women

Hemoglobin (Hgb): 13 to 17 g/dL in men/12 to 15 g/dL in women

Hematocrit (HcT): 40% to 52% in men/36% to 47% in women

Platelets: 150 to 400 units/L

White blood cell (WBCs): 4.0 to 11.0 $mm^3/\mu L$

Prothrombin time (PT): 10 to 14 seconds

Partial thromboplastin time (PTT): 25 to 35 seconds

International normalizing ratio (INR): 2 to 3

Creatine kinase: 25 to 200 U/L

Creatine kinase-MB (CK-MB): 0.4 ng/mL

Troponin: 0 to 0.4 ng/mL

Serum albumin: 3.5 to 5.0 g/dL

Blood urea nitrogen (BUN): 7 to 20 mg/dL

Creatinine (Cr): 0.5 to 1.3 mg/dL

Sodium (Na): 135 to 145 mEq/L

Potassium (K): 3.5 to 5.0 mEq/L

Magnesium (Mg): 1.5 to 2.6 mg/dL

Calcium (Ca): 8.6 to 10.4 mg/dL

Phosphorus (P): 2.7 to 4.5 mg/dL

Iron (Fe): 250 to 410 mcg/dL

Ammonia (NH_3): 30 to 70 mcg/dL

CARDIOVASCULAR DISORDERS

Assessing a Patient With a Cardiovascular Disorder

To have a better understanding of the function of the heart and mechanisms of blood flow, review the structure of the heart in your anatomy and physiology textbook. Obtain a health history for any prior conditions, surgeries, or new onset of symptoms such as chest pain. Before conducting an assessment, obtain a set of vital signs and an electrocardiogram (EKG) to see the patient baseline heart rhythm. Patients who come into the hospital with chest pain are emergent cases and must be treated immediately.

Cardiac Diagnostics

Complete Blood Count (CBC): WBC, hemoglobin, hematocrit, platelets, etc.

Comprehensive Metabolic Panel (CMP): Electrolytes and renal function such as Na, K, BUN/Cr.

Cardiac Enzymes: Creatine kinase: 25 to 200 U/L, creatine kinase MB (CK-MB): 0.4 ng/mL, and troponin: 0 to 0.4 ng/mL. Used to determine if a patient is having a myocardial infarction (MI).

Clotting Factors: Prothrombin time (PT): 10 to 14 seconds, partial thromboplastin time (PTT): 25 to 35 seconds, International normalizing ratio (INR): 2 to 3.

Electrocardiogram (EKG): Along with labs, an EKG may be ordered to obtain the patient's baseline cardiac rhythm. Abnormal EKGs can signify a heart attack or MI or other disorders. Professors love to include EKG strips on tests! Knowledge of the different cardiac rhythms is even tested on the NCLEX. A packet of cardiac strips will be provided in class; also refer to your textbook. I will not go into too much detail in this chapter. Refer to Appendix C for sample EKGs. I will explain the purpose of the EKG and its diagnostic use below:

- EKGs measure electrical conduction of the heart, but do not reflect cardiac output.
- → **The SA node in the heart controls heart rate and impulses of the heart. You can look at the SA node as being a person's pacemaker.**
- Be able to recognize the various rhythms such as normal sinus rhythm, sinus tachycardia, sinus bradycardia, atrial flutter, atrial fibrillation, ventricular fibrillation, asystole, and heart blocks. Refer to your textbook for pictures of the various rhythms. Some of these rhythms are also very critical, and the patient must be assessed and seen immediately.
- When a patient is in ventricular fibrillation, the number one treatment is defibrillation. CPR may also be administered per protocol. → **Defibrillation does not work on patients who are in asystole!** CPR is administered immediately.
- Patients with cardiac pacemakers will show a paced rhythm on the monitor. Pacemakers control the heart rhythm and are implanted in the chest wall. A shock is given if the HR is less than 50, depending on what the pacemaker is set to shock.
- → **Patients with pacemakers are advised to use caution when receiving MRIs, but recent studies have shown it is safe.**
- Antidysrhythmic or anticoagulant medications should be administered to patients who suffer from dysrhythmias.

Echocardiogram: An ultrasound used to obtain valve function in the heart.

Stress Test: Using a treadmill to increase heart rate through exercising to see the patient's cardiac response to activity.

Hypertension

Definition: Blood pressure is the force of blood exerted on the vessel walls measured in systolic and diastolic pressures. The systolic pressure represents the ejection of the blood from the heart into the arteries, and the diastolic pressure the heart at rest between beats. Blood pressure is measured using a sphygmomanometer (in simplest terms, a blood pressure cuff) or Dynamap (an electronic reading of BP). **The most accurate way to obtain a BP is by manually taking the blood pressure with a cuff and stethoscope. Electronic measurements can be slightly off.** ←

A normal blood pressure reading is anything less than 120/80 mmHg. According to the American Heart Association, anything above 120/80 to 140/80 mmHg is considered prehypertensive. Stage I hypertension is anything from 140/90 to 159/90 mmHg. Stage II hypertension is greater than 160 mmHg. Stage III, which is considered an emergency and must be treated immediately, is blood pressure that reads above 180 mmHg. A sustained hypertensive state can lead to stroke. Hypotension is the complete opposite: Anything below 100/80 mmHg is considered hypotensive. Hypotension can lead to dizziness or fainting. Report any abnormal findings to the physician immediately.

Signs and Symptoms:

Hypertension: Patients who are hypertensive may be asymptomatic and may be diagnosed during physical exams. When blood pressure remains elevated for a period of time, the patient may begin to feel symptoms of headache, increased heart rate, chest pain, sweating, vision changes, and edema. Hypertension is known as a "silent killer" when left untreated. Hypertension can lead to plaque buildup in the artery walls that can cause complications such as heart attacks or strokes if left untreated.

Hypotension: Patients who are hypotensive may experience dizziness, weakness, fatigue, sweating, or anxiety. On exam, the nurse or physician may obtain an orthostatic blood pressure reading to see if there is a rapid decrease in blood pressure when standing, a common problem. Orthostatic BP is first taken lying down, sitting upright, and then standing. If the numbers drastically change from the lying to the standing position—for example, say a patient's supine BP is 125/80 mmHg and standing BP is 95/80 mmHg—the patient is considered to have orthostatic hypertension. Use safety measures with these patients due to the risk of falls and dizziness. Patients who are postsurgical or have GI bleeds can suffer from hypotension as well.

Diagnostics: Obtain blood pressure, cholesterol levels/lipid profile to see if there is buildup of plaque in the arteries, CBC, clotting factors PT/INR, BUN/Cr for kidney function and CMP.

→ *Complications:* **A sustained elevated blood pressure can cause organ damage, coronary artery disease, stroke, retinal damage, heart attacks, and renal disease if left untreated.** Patients with blood pressure sustained above 180 mmHg may need ICU treatment or more aggressive treatment to lower the blood pressure.

Drug Therapy:

- Antihypertensive medications:
  - Beta-blockers: These include atenolol (Tenormin), propranolol (Inderal), labetalol (Trandate), metoprolol (Lopressor/Toprol XL), carvedilol (Coreg), acebutolol (Sectral), and bisoprolol (Zebeta). Beta-blockers block epinephrine and decrease the heart rate and the heart's demand for oxygen. Always obtain vital signs before administering. Do not administer if the patient is hypotensive or has a heart rate less than 60 bpm.
  - Angiotensin-converting enzyme (ACE) inhibitors: These include captopril (Capoten), lisinopril (Zestril), enalapril (Vasotec), ramipril (Altace), quinapril (Accupril), benazepril (Lotensin), and fosinopril (Monopril). ACE inhibitors dilate the blood vessels and increase blood flow, decreasing blood pressure and the amount the heart has to work to pump blood.
  - Calcium channel blockers (CCBs): These include amlodipine (Norvasc), diltiazem (Cardizem), verapamil (Calan), and nifedipine (Procardia). CCBs also dilate the blood vessels, which increases blood flow and decreases blood pressure.
  - Angiotensin receptor blockers (ARBs): These include losartan (Cozaar), olmesartan (Benicar), valsartan (Diovan), telmisartan (Micardis), candesartan (Atacand), and irbesartan (Avapro). ARBs dilate the blood vessels to decrease blood pressure. They also promote excretion of sodium and water into the urine to decrease blood pressure.

- Thiazide diuretics/loop diuretics: Hydrochlorothiazide (HCTZ) and metolazone (Zaroxolyn) are thiazide diuretics. Loop diuretics are furosemide (Lasix), bumetanide (Bumex), and toresmide (Demadex). Diuretics help release fluid through the urine, decreasing both edema and blood pressure.
- Vasodilators: These are used in the hospital, not frequently given as a home med. Vasodilators inlcude apresoline (Hydralazine) and nipride (Nitroprusside), which is given intravenously to decrease blood pressure rapidly. It is important to closely monitor these patients.
- Antiadrenergics: The one most commonly administered is clonidine (Catapres), given orally to decrease blood pressure.

Nursing Care: Patient education is very important, and treating hypertension is the key to preventing further complications. Continuous monitoring of blood pressure and regular checkups are needed. Teach patients to maintain a low-sodium diet and regularly exercise to promote a healthy lifestyle. Antihypertensive medications can cause a decrease in blood pressure, and it is important to teach the patient signs of hypotension. These medications also have a side effect of a persistent dry cough; if these symptoms occur, speak to your physician, because a change in medication may be needed. Medications are often prescribed daily in the morning or twice a day.

Congestive Heart Failure

Definition: Congestive heart failure (CHF) is an accumulation of fluid around the heart and lungs that causes a decrease in cardiac output. CHF causes fluid overload, meaning too much fluid in the lungs. Heart failure can occur on either side of the heart, which is then termed right-sided heart failure or left-sided heart failure. Each side presents with different symptoms.

Signs and Symptoms:

Right-sided heart failure: Weight gain, ascites, nausea, edema in the upper and lower extremities, and jugular vein distension (bounding pulses).

Left-sided heart failure: Cough, dusky color skin, chest pain, shortness of breath, fatigue, weakness, crackles in the lungs, wheezes, palpitations, decreased oxygen saturation, anxiety, and difficulty breathing.

Diagnostics: A lab test called ProBNP (shows the amount of fluid accumulation in the body), as well as BUN/Cr, CBC, basic metabolic panel (paying close attention to potassium levels), and a chest x-ray are obtained, and a cardiac monitor may be placed on the patient.

Complications: Respiratory distress, pulmonary edema, renal failure, cardiogenic shock, hepatomegaly, cardiac arrhythmias, and death.

Drug Therapy: These patients must be admitted to the hospital immediately for intravenous diuretics. Diuretics decrease the amount of fluids in the body by excreting sodium and potassium. IV furosemide (Lasix) is often administered to patients with CHF in a hospital setting. Other diuretics such as spironolactone (Aldactone) are administered orally to treat patients who suffer from chronic CHF. ACE inhibitors and CCBs are also used to treat CHF.

Nebulizer treatments may be administered to facilitate breathing and help with congestion.

Nursing Care: Assess the patient's respiratory status, oxygen saturation, and mentation, and listen to the lungs. If the patient is having difficulty breathing and you hear crackles in the lungs, the patient may be experiencing fluid overload, and an IV diuretic may be needed; call the doctor immediately. O_2 may be placed on the patient to maintain oxygen saturation levels. Discontinue intravenous fluids, and monitor intake and output. Output should be documented every shift, to ensure that the fluid is being excreted properly. A fluid restriction may be ordered. Place the patient in high Fowler's position at a 45° to 90° angle to facilitate breathing. Daily weights are needed to monitor the fluid overload. Elevate upper and lower extremities if edematous.

Angina Pectoris

Definition: Severe chest pain caused by sclerosis of the arteries and myocardial ischemia. Do not confuse angina pectoris with an MI. Angina is chest pain that is relieved by medication, and there is no permanent damage to the myocardial tissue. Angina is caused by an imbalance of oxygen supply and demand. An MI involves actual cell death.

Signs and Symptoms: Chest pain, chest pressure, sweating, palpitations, dizziness, anxiety, and dyspnea.

Diagnostics: For patients with angina pectoris, an MI must first be ruled out. An EKG, cardiac enzymes, troponin levels, and a chest x-ray should be obtained.

Complications: Myocardial infarction and dysrhythmias.

Drug Therapy: Nitroglycerin, a vasodilator, is given sublingually and controls ischemic pain. Always wear gloves to administer nitro because it can cause severe hypotension. Assess the patient's blood pressure before administering nitro. Give the first tablet sublingually; then, if the pain persists in 5 minutes, give another tablet. Continue to assess blood pressure. A total of three tablets can be given. Intravenous morphine sulfate is used to control pain if not relieved by nitroglycerin. Beta adrenergic receptors are given to decrease cardiac output. Anticoagulants are given to prevent pulmonary emboli. If angina persists, surgery may be needed. A percutaneous cardiac intervention (stent) or coronary bypass graft may be performed.

Storage of nitroglycerin is also important. It should be placed in a cool and dark place. Light can decrease its effectiveness. Gloves should be worn when administering nitroglycerin. ←

Nursing Care: When a patient presents with chest pain, it is important to distinguish whether the patient is having an MI or true angina through diagnostic testing. Once an MI is ruled out, treatment for angina is started. Administer oxygen to the patient. Place patient on strict bed rest. Continue to assess blood pressure, due to the risk of hypotension. Monitor vital signs frequently. If surgery is done, use surgical precautions. Patient education is important.

Myocardial Infarction

Definition: Myocardial infarction (MI) occurs when ischemia of the ventricles causes a disruption of blood flow and oxygen to the heart. A patient presenting with an MI is considered an emergent situation.

Signs and Symptoms: Chest pain that radiates to the shoulder or back, nausea, vomiting, increased blood pressure, pulmonary edema, dizziness, anxiety, weakness, fatigue, shortness of breath, increased pulse, elevated ST on an EKG, and elevated troponins.

Diagnostics: EKG, CBC, CMP, PT/INR, BUN/Cr, cardiac enzymes, CK-MB, troponins, cardiac monitoring, and chest

→ x-ray. **CK rises within 4 to 6 hours of an MI, peaks in 24 to 72 hours, and last for 3 days. Troponin levels rise within 4 to 6 hours and remain high for 2 weeks. Lactate dehydrogenase increases in MI, and levels last for 3 days.** If these labs are elevated, an MI must be ruled out immediately.

Complications: Cardiogenic shock, heart failure, pulmonary embolism, and death if left untreated.

Drug Therapy: An MI is a critical event, and drug therapy needs to be rapidly administered. Morphine/nitroglycerin is given to relieve pain. Oxygen is administered to maintain oxygen levels. Aspirin or clopidogrel (Plavix) is given as an anticoagulant. Antidysrhythmics are given to prevent fatal arrhythmias. Fibrinolytic therapy may be needed to prevent blood clots and dissolve plaque in the arteries, to increase perfusion and decrease ischemia to the heart. → **Fibrinolytic therapy is effective within 6 hours of an MI.** Intravenous fluids are administered.

Nursing Care:

An MI is considered an emergent situation; these patients are often placed in the ICU until stable. Administer medications as ordered. Administer oxygen to patient. Monitor vital signs closely. Patient is placed on continuous cardiac monitoring. Serial labs of troponin levels are performed. Keep patient calm and decrease anxiety. Patient activity is limited and patients are placed on strict bed rest. Lifestyle changes such as diet, exercise, smoking cessation, and regularly scheduled checkups are discussed.

These patients may require surgery such as percutaneous transluminal coronary angioplasty (PTCA), and coronary bypass graft or stent placement may be needed.

Coronary Artery Disease

Definition: In coronary artery disease, plaque builds up on the blood vessel walls, leading to narrowing or blockage in the artery known as *atherosclerosis.* It is commonly caused by high cholesterol, smoking, a high-fat diet, and hypertension.

Signs and Symptoms: These include poor circulation, headache, dizziness, and angina, but patients may appear asymptomatic.

Diagnostics: These include CBC, CMP, PT/INR, cardiac enzymes, EKG, stress test, chest x-ray, cardiac angiography, and cardiac catheterization. Lipid profile total cholesterol should be less than 200. LDL is greater than 160 mg/dL, and HDL is less than 40 mg/dL.

Complications: Heart failure, dysrhythmias, MI, and death if left untreated.

Drug Therapy: Antilipidemic medications, such as atorvastatin (Lipitor) and simvastatin (Zocor), are administered to decrease cholesterol levels and calcium nitrates. Calcium channel blockers are also administered. Treat any underlying cause. Cardiac catheterization or stent placement may be needed to facilitate adequate blood flow. Coronary bypass surgery may be needed if sclerosis is severe.

Nursing Care: Administer medication as ordered. Patient teaching is performed to encourage maintenance of a healthy diet, regular exercise, and smoking cessation. Continue to monitor cholesterol levels. If surgery is needed, provide preoperative and postoperative teaching.

Deep Vein Thrombosis

Definition: This refers to thrombus formation (blood clot) in one or more deep veins in the body, commonly in the lower extremities or groin. Blood clots are dangerous because they can break off and travel to different parts of the body such as the lungs.

Signs and Symptoms: Edema or swelling in the extremity. The affected area is warm, edematous, tender, and reddened. Positive Homan's sign (dorsiflexion causes extreme pain).

Diagnostics: **Ultrasound of the affected extremity**, Doppler, CT scan, or x-ray. Lab work such as PTT, PT, and INR will need to be obtained. ←

Complications: Pulmonary embolism, leg ulcerations, and venous insufficiency.

Drug Therapy: Anticoagulants such as Lovenox, heparin, Xeralto, Coumadin, or Arixtra. Anti-inflammatory medications such as Toradol to control inflammation and pain. Fibrinolytic medications may also be needed.

Nursing Care:

Once the ultrasound confirms there is a DVT, the patient is immediately started on an anticoagulant. It is important to teach the patient about the risk of bleeding. Due to the increased risk of bleeding, patients should be careful when shaving. Instruct patients to use an electric razor. Because there is also an increased risk of bruising, instruct patients to use caution when walking. For any invasive procedures, anticoagulants must be stopped for 48 hours prior to any procedures. Elevate the affected extremity. Apply a warm compress to the site to decrease inflammation. If there is a blood clot in an upper extremity, make sure to put a "restricted extremity" armband on that extremity. No blood pressure or labs must be taken from that arm. Complete bed rest is ordered. If there is a blood clot in a lower extremity, do not apply sequential compression devices (SCDs) or thromboembolic deterrent devices (TEDs) on the affected leg. Continue to monitor clotting factors.

Surgical procedures such as venous thrombectomy may need to be performed.

Peripheral Artery Disease

Definition: In this condition, there is a decrease in the blood flow and oxygenation to the extremities caused by atherosclerosis.

Signs and Symptoms: Bilateral leg pain, darkening of the skin, tingling, cyanosis, weak pulse, and poor circulation to the lower extremities.

Diagnostics: Ultrasound and angiography. Clotting factors and CBC also need to be obtained (paying close attention for signs of infection).

Complications: Necrosis, infection, and ulcerations. In advanced stages, amputation of the extremity is necessary.

Drug Therapy: Anticoagulants, antihyperlipidemics, antiplatelet, and antihypertensives are needed.

Nursing Care:

Control cholesterol levels and blood pressure, along with diabetes management, if needed, with the ordered medications. Maintain a low-fat/sodium diet. Administer skin care or wound care if ulcers are present. Avoid applying extreme temperatures to the extremity. Assess pulses, use Doppler stethoscope if unable to palpate. If the patient is a smoker, offer smoking cessation. Provide comfort.

Surgical procedures such as peripheral endarterectomy (removal of plaque in the artery), bypass graft, or amputation, may be required, depending on the severity. Nonsurgical measures such as angioplasty or stent may be placed to open up the artery walls and allow better blood flow. If surgery is needed, provide preoperative and postoperative instructions.

Chronic Venous Insufficiency

Definition: Insufficient blood flow to the veins in the legs, causing ulcers or cellulitis.

Signs and Symptoms: Redness, edema, itching, flaking, ulcerations, pain, and skin that appears tough and dry.

Diagnostics: Obtain an ultrasound to rule out DVT.

Complications: Ulcerations.

Drug Therapy: Antibiotics are commonly administered.

Nursing Care: Dressing changes and wound care for the affected site. Administer antibiotics as ordered. Decrease risks of clots. Elevate extremity. SCDs are applied to increase blood flow, but use precaution when applying to the affected extremities. Assess pulses.

Endocarditis

Definition: Endocarditis is infection and inflammation of the valves and endocardium of the heart. It is caused by bacterial infection or vegetation.

Signs and Symptoms: **Fever, chills, weakness, fatigue, weight loss, murmurs, Janeway lesion (flat red spots on the palms and soles, Osler's nodes on hands/feet, and red blotches on the skin).** ←

Diagnostics: EKG, echocardiogram, CBC, and blood cultures.

Complications: Embolism and heart failure.

Drug Therapy: Aggressive antibiotic therapy.

Nursing Care: Assess for complications such as emboli. Administer long-term antibiotics and educate the patients on their use. Ensure cardiac monitoring. Bed rest is ordered. Continue to monitor for signs of heart failure. Patients who are IV drug users are at the highest risk of endocarditis, and the risks of using drugs should be taught to the patient. Patients should avoid exercise or strenuous activity.

Pericarditis

Definition: Pericarditis is infection and inflammation of the pericardium of the heart.

Signs and Symptoms: Chest pain, respiration changes, fever, shortness of breath, and signs of heart failure.

Diagnostics: EKG, CBC, WBC, chest x-ray, and increased C-reactive protein (CRP).

Complications: Fluid in the pericardium that is left untreated can lead to cardiac tamponade. **Signs of cardiac tamponade are muffled heart sounds, increased heart rate and respirations, and jugular vein distension.** ←

Drug Therapy: Nonsteroidal anti-inflammatory (NSAIDs), corticosteroids, antibiotics, cardiac glycoside (Digoxin), and, possibly, a diuretic.

Nursing Care: Provide comfort and monitor for levels of pain and anxiety. Administer medications as ordered. Assess and monitor for complications.

Cardiac Valve Disorders

Hang in there! We are almost through cardiac disorders. Last, but not least, we will discuss valve disorders of the heart. You will be responsible for knowing the five main diseases, but will not need to go into too much detail. These disorders are caused by infective endocarditis, ischemia, or congenital heart disease. Diagnostic testing, such as an echocardiogram, EKG, or stress test, is used to distinguish the valve disorders. Explanations of the five main disorders of the mitral valve and aortic valves are listed here:

1. *Mitral valve stenosis*: Calcification of the left atrium of the heart is the most common of the valve disorders. Causes pulmonary congestion. Symptoms are shortness of breath, fatigue, cardiac murmur, palpitations, and emboli. Medications such as diuretics, antibiotics, and anticoagulants are given.
2. *Mitral valve regurgitation*: Blood flow is forced into the left atrium of the heart. Causes pulmonary edema, abnormal pulse, and symptoms of heart failure. Medications such as diuretics, antibiotics, ACE inhibitors, cardiac glycoside (Digoxin), and anticoagulants are given.
3. *Mitral valve prolapse*: A prolapse occurs in the left atrium of the heart. Symptoms are heart murmurs, chest pain, and arrhythmias. Antibiotics and beta-blockers are commonly administered.
4. *Aortic valve stenosis*: Calcification of the aortic valve. Symptoms are dizziness, vertigo, angina, shortness of breath, fatigue, and murmurs. Rheumatic heart disease can cause stenosis; it is important to treat the underlying cause. Medications such as antibiotics, cardiac glycosides, beta-blockers, and diuretics may be administered.
5. *Aortic valve regurgitation*: Blood flow is forced back into the aortic valve. Shortness of breath is usually the first symptom. Diuretics are often administered to relieve symptoms of fluid overload.

Nursing Care: Monitor for complications. Monitor vital signs. Ensure continuous cardiac monitoring. Administer medications as ordered. Surgical procedures such as open heart surgery for valve replacement or cardiac catheterization may be needed. Limit activity.

Cardiac Arrhythmias

You will be required to know the various cardiac arrhythmias. Some examples of the common rhythms seen are included in Appendix C. I will explain the most common arrhythmias here:

- Normal sinus rhythm: Regular and heart rate is 60 to 100 bpm.
- Atrial fibrillation: No "P" waves. Controlled rate of 60 to 100 bpm or can be uncontrolled with a rate greater than 100 bpm. Patients are at risk for clots and need to be put on anticoagulants to prevent thrombosis. Medications such as Coumadin or Xeralto can be given. Also, patients receive an ablation to treat A-fib.
- Sinus bradycardia: Heart rate below 60 bpm. Hold all blood pressure medication when the pulse is less than 60 bpm. If the heart rate does not increase, a pacemaker may be needed.
- Sinus tachycardia: A heart rate greater than 100 bpm. Medications such as Lopressor may be given.
- Ventricular fibrillation: Very rapid and disorganized. Patient is unresponsive. Initiate CPR. Defibrillation is needed.

RESPIRATORY DISORDERS

Assessing a Patient With Respiratory Disorders

Review the anatomy and physiology of the lungs in your textbook. Obtain a health history from the patient. Assess both any new symptoms and chronic disorders the patient may have. Obtain a set of vital signs and oxygen (O_2) level. If saturation levels are below 92%, oxygen may be administered to the patient through a nasal cannula at 2 L. Any patients who are experiencing shortness of breath or any change in respirations are considered emergencies and must be seen immediately. Remember that maintaining an airway is always important and takes priority!

Respiratory Diagnostics

Lab Work: CBC, CMP, ProBNP, blood cultures, and D-dimer are typically assessed.

Chest x-ray

Pulse Oximetry: Measured by placing a sensor on the finger. Normal range is anything above 95% to 100%. If nail polish or acrylic nails are present on a female patient, this may affect the reading and must be removed.

Arterial Blood Gases: Refer to the chart in the previous chapter for values.

Sputum Cultures: Sputum taken from the patient and tested for specific organisms.

Pulmonary Function Tests (PFTs): Measure lung volume and airflow.

Bronchoscopy: Procedure in which the bronchi are observed and the upper airway, including the larynx, trachea, and bronchi, is visualized.

Computed Tomography Angiogram (CTA) of the Chest: Visualization of the chest for any congestion, fluid, masses, or blood clots.

Pulmonary Angiogram: Dye is injected into the pulmonary arteries to determine whether a pulmonary embolism is present.

Mantoux Skin Test: Purified protein derivative (PPD) is used to diagnose tuberculosis. A positive reaction to the PPD test is noted when a patient has been exposed to *Mycobacterium tuberculosis*; results are available in 48 to 72 hours.

Lung Biopsy: Obtaining a tissue sample from the lung to diagnose disorders such as lung cancer.

Thoracentesis: Removal of fluid from the pleural cavity.

Lung (V/Q) Scan: Dye is injected and is used to determine whether there are any defects in blood perfusion in the lungs. It is used to diagnose pulmonary embolism.

Asthma

Definition: Chronic inflammation and muscle contractions of the lungs that are often caused by triggers or allergens. Triggers can be stress, food, medications, exercise, infections, mold, or dust.

Signs and Symptoms: Wheezing, chest tightness, cough, increased mucus secretions, diminished lung sounds, decreased oxygen saturation levels, anxiety, and use of accessory muscles to breathe.

Diagnostics: Pulse oximetry, symptoms, PFTs, ABGs, and allergy skin testing.

Complications: Status asthmaticus and respiratory distress.

Drug Therapy: Beta2-adrenergic agonists such as albuterol. → **Albuterol is administered as first-line treatment, because it is fast acting, and is termed a rescue inhaler.** Inhaled corticosteroids, oral anti-inflammatories, and leukotriene modifiers (Singulair) are ordered. Long-term corticosteroids are administered to control asthma, and bronchodilators such as

Serevent, anticholinergics such as Atrovent, and expectorants such as Mucinex may be used. Oxygen may be administered.

Nursing Care: For patients experiencing acute shortness of breath and wheezing, assess oxygenation and respiratory status immediately. Monitor oxygen levels and administer oxygen as needed. Obtain ABGs and other labs. Place patient on strict bed rest. Common side effects of inhalers are tremors, nervousness, and increased heart rate; and patients need to be educated about medications. Avoid the use of fragrance, flowers, and other triggers while in the hospital. Monitor activity level. Patients should sit in high Fowler's position to facilitate better breathing. **Peak flow meters are often given to patients to allow them to measure the highest airflow during a forced expiration. The results help measure the severity of asthma.** ←

Hypoxia

Definition: Decreased oxygen levels caused by heart failure, ischemia, respiratory disorders, or anemia.

Signs and Symptoms: Restlessness, shortness of breath, low oxygen levels, anxiety, increased heart rate, and altered mental status.

Diagnostics: ABGs and oxygen saturation levels.

Complications: Chronic hypoxia or respiratory distress.

Drug Therapy: Treat the underlying cause. Administer oxygen through a mask or nasal cannula. Bilevel positive airway pressure (BiPAP) therapy may be needed.

Nursing Care: Monitor oxygen levels. Encourage deep breathing and cough. Place patients in high Fowler's position. Administer chest physiotherapy and oxygen therapy as ordered. Monitor for complications.

Chronic Obstructive Pulmonary Disorder (COPD)

Definition: A progressive and chronic obstruction of airflow, this condition encompasses chronic bronchitis, emphysema, and other disorders. Smoking is the most common cause. Patients are often admitted to the hospital for COPD exacerbations.

Signs and Symptoms: Shortness of breath, hypoxia, cough, diminished breath sounds, barrel chest, fatigue, anxiety, and anorexia.

Diagnostics: Oxygen levels, ABGs (respiratory acidosis), chest x-ray, and PFTs.

➔ *Complications:* **Pneumonia, GERD, acute respiratory failure, and cor pulmonale (right-sided heart failure).**

Drug Therapy: Bronchodilators, corticosteroids, antibiotics, expectorants, and oxygen therapy. Nebulizers and steroids such as Solumedrol or prednisone are given as first-line treatments.

Nursing Care: Maintain oxygen saturation levels. Administer medications as ordered. A respiratory therapist will also assess the patient frequently. Chest physiotherapy is performed to help break up secretions. Teach the patient to conserve energy, and schedule periods of rest. Smoking cessation assistance should be provided. ➔ **Monitor glucose levels, as steroids tend to increase blood glucose levels.** Observe for and prevent complications that may arise.

Pneumonia

Definition: Pneumonia is inflammation of the lung tissues and alveoli. Pneumonia can be caused by infection, aspiration of fluid or food, and accumulation of fluid. It can be viral or bacterial (*Streptococcus pneumoniae, Mycoplasma pneumoniae,* or *Staphylococcus aureus).*

Signs and Symptoms: Fever, cough, chest pain, chest tightness, increased secretions, chills, diminished breath sounds, wheezing, crackles, and hypoxia.

Diagnostics: Labs, chest x-ray, PFTs, ABGs, blood cultures, and sputum culture. ➔ **Antibiotics are often administered once a sputum culture is obtained.** Chest x-ray will show pleural effusion or infiltrates when pneumonia is present.

Complications: Respiratory failure and sepsis

Drug Therapy: Antibiotics, bronchodilators, analgesics, steroids, and antipyretics.

Nursing Care: Oxygen therapy. Monitor vital signs, and closely monitor the patient's temperature. Patients should be placed in high Fowler's position to facilitate breathing. Nebulizer treatments are administered. Monitor lab work, including WBC and glucose levels. Place sterile specimen cup at bedside for patient to use for sputum culture. The first sputum of the morning is best. Maintain nutrition and hydration. When the patient is treated for pneumonia and no longer exhibits symptoms, a pneumonia vaccine is administered to prevent further cases.

Pleural Effusion

Definition: This is the accumulation of fluid in the pleural space of the chest. Pleural effusion is often caused by CHF, pneumonia, TB, pulmonary emboli, or lung cancer.

Signs and Symptoms: **Pulmonary congestion, chest pain, crackles, edema, shortness of breath, and decreased breath sounds.** ←

Diagnostics: Chest x-ray, CT of the chest, and culture of pleural fluid.

Complications: If left untreated, respiratory distress or worsening of symptoms.

Drug Therapy: Diuretics are used to remove fluid from the lungs. Antipyretics are used if a fever is present.

Nursing Care: Monitor respiratory status. Administer oxygen as needed. Administer medications as ordered. A thoracentesis or chest tube may be placed to remove fluid from the lungs. Assess chest tube or thoracentesis site. Assess lung sounds throughout the shift, monitoring for any changes.

Pulmonary Edema

Definition: Pulmonary edema is accumulation of fluid in the lungs. It can be caused by heart failure or fluid overload.

Signs and Symptoms: Shortness of breath, crackles heard on auscultation, edema, restlessness, cough, tachycardia, and wet breath sounds.

Diagnostics: **Chest x-ray and ProBNP to assess for heart failure and fluid overload.** ←

Complications: Respiratory distress.

Drug Therapy: Diuretics, oxygen therapy, patients may require BiPAP, vasodilators, and mechanical ventilation in severe cases.

Nursing Care: Assess vital signs and oxygen. Maintain a patent airway. Place patients in high Fowler's position. Complete bed rest is ordered. Administer medications as ordered. Cardiac monitoring may be ordered. Continue to monitor potassium. Fluid restriction will be needed. Monitor strict intake and output.

Tuberculosis

Definition: TB is an infectious disease spread by the organism *Mycobacterium tuberculosis*, transferred through respiratory droplets.

Signs and Symptoms: Fatigue, anorexia, cough, chest pain, night sweats, chills, crackles, and hemoptysis.

Diagnostics: Chest x-ray, Mantoux test, QuantiFERON-TB (QFT) blood test, and acid-fast bacilli (AFBs). → **AFBs are sputum cultures that test positive when a patient has active tuberculosis.** Three sputum cultures need to test positive to make a diagnosis of TB. If the tests are positive, a chest x-ray is done to confirm the results. The patient is then immediately placed on treatment and airborne precautions. Sputum culture is checked every 2 weeks until negative.

Complications: Pneumonia and worsening of infection.

Drug Therapy: Broad-spectrum antibiotics are administered to patients diagnosed with TB: (a) isoniazid (INH), (b) rifampin (Rifadin), (c) pyrazinamide (PZA), (d) rifabutin (Mycobutin), and (e) ethambutol (Myambutol). Refer to Chapter 5 for further details on these medications, including common side effects. Antipyretics are administered to control temperatures.

Nursing Care: Once a patient exhibits symptoms of TB, he or she is placed in a negative pressure room and droplet precautions are applied. An N95 mask must be worn at all times when in contact with the patient. N95 masks are worn at all times when in contact with the patient. → **Patients are placed in a negative pressure room and placed on droplet precautions.** Medications are usually taken for 6 to 12 months with the sputum culture checked every 2 to 4 weeks. Provide adequate nutrition and hydration. Monitor vital signs and temperature. Provide periods of rest and limit activity. Visitors may be prohibited, especially children, while patients are on droplet precautions. Adhere to strict hand-washing guidelines and standard precautions.

Influenza

Definition: Commonly known as the "flu," influenza is an infectious disease caused by the influenza virus.

Signs and Symptoms: Fever, chills, cough, fatigue, body aches, headache, and nasal congestion.

Diagnostics: Nasal swab to test for influenza A or influenza B.

Complications: If left untreated, symptoms can worsen, leading to pneumonia, and for patients who are immunocompromised, further complications can arise.

Drug Therapy: Antivirals such as oseltamivir (Tamiflu) or zanamivir (Relenza). M2 inhibitors such as amantadine (Symmetrel) and rimantadine (Flumadine) are also used to treat the flu.

Nursing Care: Patients who present with symptoms of the flu are placed on airborne precautions and should wear a mask when exposed to others to prevent infection. A mask must be worn when taking care of these patients. To prevent infection, flu vaccines are administered yearly. Monitor vital signs and temperature. Administer antivirals as ordered.

Ebola

Definition: This infection is caused by the Ebola virus, which has caused recurring outbreaks of disease in western African countries. Ebola is spread through bodily secretions (mucus, sweat, tears, etc.). According to the World Health Organization, in 2013, the largest outbreak occurred and is an ongoing epidemic. Cases in the United States began to appear, and Ebola precautions were put in place immediately.

Signs and Symptoms: The development of symptoms or incubation period is 2 to 21 days. Symptoms are flulike initially but quickly escalate to include fevers, cough, severe headache, joint pain, chest pain, hypotension, shortness of breath, bleeding, hemoptysis, and bloody stools.

Diagnostics: Lab work and ELISA test.

Complications: Respiratory distress, sepsis, and death.

Drug Therapy: Antivirals such as Ribavirin are used to treat Ebola. Antipyretics are used to control temperatures. Administer intravenous fluids to hydrate patient.

Nursing Care: Patients who exhibit symptoms of Ebola are placed in an isolation room immediately. Protective wear is put on at once, and the CDC must be called for further instructions. These patients must stay in the isolated area until further instructions from the CDC. It is important to ask patients who present with symptoms of Ebola if they have traveled out of the country recently.

Pulmonary Embolism

Definition: This is a blockage in the pulmonary artery caused by a blood clot. It often occurs when a clot that is formed elsewhere in the body travels to the lungs. This is an emergent situation!

Signs and Symptoms: Shortness of breath, cough, blood-tinged sputum, chest pain, crackles, anxiety, and increased respirations.

Diagnostics: **CTA of the chest, D-dimer, V/Q scan, and clotting factors.** ←

Complications: Sudden death if the clot is large and left untreated.

Drug Therapy: Anticoagulants are administered. Patients are often put on a continuous heparin drip with frequent monitoring of PTT, PT, and INR levels. Thrombolytics may be administered. Medications to decrease anxiety may also be given.

Nursing Care: Patients who present with symptoms of a PE must be seen and diagnosed immediately. Maintain airway and vital signs. Administer anticoagulants once a diagnosis is made. Ensure strict bed rest and administer oxygen therapy. Adequate hydration and nutrition is needed.

Acute Respiratory Distress Syndrome (ARDS)

Definition: Acute respiratory distress syndrome is increased fluid in the interstitial space and alveoli of the lungs causing respiratory acidosis. ARDS is caused by pneumonia, chest injury, shock, or embolism. This is considered an emergent situation, and the patient must be seen immediately.

Signs and Symptoms: Hypoxia, shortness of breath, fatigue, decreased oxygen levels, chest pain, increased heart rate, confusion, use of accessory muscles, and cyanosis. Patient appears to be in distress.

Diagnostics: Oxygen saturation level, chest x-ray, ABGs, and CT scan of the chest.

Complications: Pulmonary collapse, respiratory failure, and shock.

Drug Therapy: Antibiotics, oxygen therapy, IV hydration, vasopressors, pulmonary vasodilators, and diuretics may be needed. Always treat the underlying cause.

Nursing Care: Maintain a patent airway, and assess respiratory status. Maintain oxygenation. Patient may be placed on mechanical ventilation or need an endotracheal intubation to improve ventilation. Positive end-expiratory pressure (PEEP) is used to improve ventilation as well. These patients are often placed in the ICU and are closely monitored. Administer medications as ordered.

Acute Respiratory Failure

Definition: This is the lack of oxygen to the lungs, which is most often due to the increase of fluid in the airspace. It causes a decrease in oxygen in the blood and an increase in carbon dioxide.

Signs and Symptoms: Cyanosis, tachycardia, decreased O_2 levels, increased BP, confusion, and restlessness. → **Change in mental status is a first sign that there is a lack of oxygen.**

Diagnostics: CT of the chest and ABGs.

Complications: Death can occur if left untreated.

Drug Therapy: Oxygen therapy, bronchodilators, corticosteroids, or mechanical ventilation may be needed.

Nursing Care:

This is an emergent situation, and patients must be seen at once. Maintain a patent airway and O_2 saturation levels. Patient may be placed on PEEP or intubated. Once off the ventilator, assess patient's O_2 levels. Maintain adequate hydration and nutrition. Provide rest, and place restrictions on strenuous activity.

Continue to closely monitor vital signs and signs of infection.

Artificial Airways/Chest Tubes/Ventilators

Focus on this section in detail. I will describe the most frequently tested and important information. Use this section as study aid to your textbook and class notes. You will be required to know the different artificial airways and nursing care for all. Just a little heads-up: The information in this section was often included on tests.

Endotracheal Intubation

Definition: Placement of an endotracheal tube through the mouth or nose into the trachea to maintain a patent airway. This is used in emergencies on patients with respiratory distress or respiratory failure. **Oral intubation is the first choice in a critical situation because of the size of the tube and the rapid opening of the airway.** Nasal intubation would be the second choice if oral **intubation** was not accessible. Remember, never use nasal intubation for a patient who has a facial injury or one in whom the oral airway is obstructed. ←

Intubation Procedure/Nursing Care: A physician performs the insertion of the endotracheal tube with the assistance of the nurse. Prepare all equipment for the insertion. Sedate the patient and apply soft restraints to keep the patient from pulling out the tube. Keep the head of the bed flat and suction equipment nearby. A crash cart may be needed at the bedside. As the tube is being inserted, the nurse's role is to provide oxygen to the patient using an Ambu bag. The patient receives 100% of oxygen for 3 to 5 minutes. After insertion, the cuff is inflated while on the ventilator. Assess for chest symmetry and breath sounds every 2 hours. ABGs are evaluated every 20 to 30 minutes. **At the end of the procedure, a chest x-ray is done to ensure proper placement of the tube.** Intubated patients are closely monitored in the ICU. ←

Tracheostomy

Definition: This is a surgical opening of the trachea to maintain an open airway. Tracheostomy can be used for long-term or short-term airway assistance. A fenestrated tracheostomy is used with a ventilator and without. The nursing role in caring for a patient with a tracheostomy is to remove secretions, provide trach care, and maintain the airway.

Nursing Care: Using sterile technique, it is important to clean the tracheostomy site. The tracheotomy tube is secured with ties. When cleaning the trach, apply new ties before removing the old ones. Removing the ties before can cause the trach to move, causing a loss of airway patency or distress. If the tracheostomy tube is accidentally removed, hold the stoma open with a hemostat until the physician arrives to place a new tube. Always maintain a patent airway and monitor oxygen levels.

Suctioning an Artificial Airway: Patients with artificial airways tend to build up secretions that they are unable to cough up on their own; these must be suctioned to clear the airway. First, auscultate lung sounds and monitor O_2 levels. Suctioning must be done in a sterile field and performed effectively to avoid complications. Explain the procedure to the patient and what to expect. If the patient has a stoma, at times the patient can self-suction.

Refer to your textbook for the exact procedure used to suction the artificial airway, and look at the images provided to gain a better understanding. → **When suctioning, the suction device should be turned on for only about 10 to 15 seconds; do not suction longer than this as doing so can compromise the patient's airway and cause a change in heart rate.** Complications of suctioning are hypoxia, respiratory distress, and damage to the airway.

Ventilators

To be honest, I was not tested much on ventilators. The three most common types are explained below.

Positive end-expiratory pressure (PEEP): It is used to maintain pressure in the alveoli of the lungs during exhalation. Ventilator settings are ordered by the physician. PEEP can cause a decrease in blood pressure.

Continuous positive airway pressure (CPAP): It is used for patients who are able to breathe spontaneously and provides a continuous flow of air. These patients do not require the ICU; CPAP can be used at the bedside or provided through the nasal cannula. CPAP is commonly used for patients with sleep apnea.

Bilevel positive airway pressure (BiPAP): This is a noninvasive type of ventilation used via face mask to deliver airflow; it differs from CPAP in that it can deliver periodic airflow instead of the continuous flow provided with CPAP.

Now you can take a deep breath! We are all finished with respiratory disorders. Hope all this information isn't causing you to experience respiratory distress.

NEUROLOGICAL DISORDERS

Assessing a Patient With Neurological Disorders

Review the anatomy and physiology of the central nervous system in your textbook. Obtain a health history from the patient. Assess any new symptoms as well as chronic neurological disorders the patient may have. Also review the cranial nerves from Chapter 2. Remember that when assessing the patient's mental status and performing the exam, culture, language, and age will affect the exam. The Glasgow Coma Scale is used to assess the neurological status of a patient:

- Eyes open: Check whether the patient can open eyes on command, and whether pupils are equal, round, and react to light.
- Verbal response: Check the patient's ability to state self, place, and year, and to answer questions appropriately. This part of the exam is used to assess pain, as well.
- Motor response: Check the patient's ability to follow commands. Also check flexion and strength of the upper and lower extremities.

An interpreter may be used to conduct this exam if the patient does not speak English. Keep in mind that older patients with an underlying problem such as dementia or Alzheimer's disease may score poorly on the scale. Neurological assessments are done on all patients. If there are any acute changes, call the physician immediately. Stroke is a common neurological emergency and must be treated immediately. We will go over the signs and symptoms of a stroke in this chapter.

Neurological Diagnostics

Magnetic Resonance Imaging (MRI): This test uses radio waves to produce images of the body. It is able to show tumors, blood vessels, and masses, and can be done with or without contrast.

Computerized Axial Tomography (CAT scan): This test uses x-ray images to dissect sections of the brain. It is able to show hemorrhage, tumors, edema, or fluid in the brain.

Electroencephalography (EEG): This test is used to measure activity in the brain by means of electrodes applied to the head. It is also used to diagnose seizures.

Lumbar Puncture: Spinal fluid is extracted from the spine at the level of L4 to L5 using a needle to aspirate the fluid. Lumbar puncture is used to diagnose meningitis or to determine if there is glucose in the spinal fluid.

Cerebral Angiogram: Cerebral blood flow is viewed by injecting dye through a catheter and gently inserting the catheter into the femoral artery to view blood flow.

Stroke

Definition: A disruption of blood flow causing interruptions in the neurological system and brain function. Also known as a cerebrovascular accident, a stroke can be caused by a hemorrhage, clot, or ischemic attack. Transient ischemic attacks (TIAs) present differently than a complete stroke.

Signs and Symptoms of TIA: Blurred vision, unsteady gait, numbness or tingling of an extremity, and slurred speech can occur. These symptoms and signs can last for several days. An MRI is used to determine if the patient is experiencing a TIA.

Signs and Symptoms of a Hemorrhagic or an Embolic Stroke:

→ **A right-sided brain injury affects the left side of the body, and a left-sided brain injury affects the right side of the body. A right-sided brain injury presents with left-sided weakness or paralysis, drooping of the face, headache, slurred speech, sensory changes, and difficulty with short-term memory or communication. A left-sided brain injury presents with right-sided weakness, right-sided face drooping, visual changes, depression, aphasia, and difficulty communicating.**

→ **Patients who experience a subarachnoid hemorrhage have distinctive symptoms, which they describe as the "worst headache of their life."**

Diagnostics: MRI or CT scan of the brain. Labs such as PT, PTT, INR.

Complications: Permanent paralysis, weakness, seizure, and death if left untreated.

Drug Therapy: Thrombolytic or fibrinolytic therapy (tissue plasminogen activator) can be used for nonhemorrhagic strokes within 3 to 4.5 hours of a stroke. Do not give patients with a subarachnoid hemorrhage fibrinolytic therapy. Diagnostics are used to determine the type of stroke. Once a stroke is diagnosed, a "stroke alert" is made. Anticoagulants are prescribed for thrombic strokes. Osmotic diuretics are used to relieve pressure in the brain. **Anticoagulants, aspirin, antiepileptics, and IV fluids are commonly used to treat strokes.** ←

Surgical Measures: Angioplasty (stent placed in the carotid artery), carotid endarterectomy (removal of plaque in the carotid arteries), and craniotomy if needed.

Nursing Care: Maintain a patent airway, and make sure the patient is not in respiratory distress. Assess airway, breathing, mental status, and vital signs. Prevention of strokes is key. The nurse's role is to first be aware of a stroke, assess signs of increased cranial pressure, identify the type of stroke, and administer medications as quickly as possible. Patients are kept in the ICU during the acute stages. A Foley catheter may be placed for adequate output records, and patients may be incontinent during the acute stages of the stroke. For patients who suffer from dysphagia, aspiration precautions need to be in place. Swallow and gag reflex needs to be assessed before patients can start eating. Thickened liquids and pureed foods may be needed. Patients may also experience weakness and paralysis on one side of their body, so it is important to maintain safety for these patients. Physical therapy and occupational therapy may be ordered to help regain strength and movement. Provide emotional support, because this period is difficult for both patients and families to cope with. Continue to conduct neuro checks every 2 to 4 hours, check vital signs every hour, and check respiratory status frequently. Be sure to report any changes or critical findings to the physician immediately.

Seizures and Epilepsy

Definition: A disruption of neurons in the brain that can be caused by trauma to the brain, tumors, infections, substance withdrawal, and/or other etiology.

Types: There are two main types of seizures: partial and generalized. Partial seizures are subdivided into two types, namely, simple partial and complex partial. The second type, generalized seizures, can be tonic-clonic, absence, or myoclonic.

Signs and Symptoms:

Simple Partial Seizures: These occur in one specific area and produce a tingling sensation in the area. Other symptoms include jerking in the area, increased heart rate, and abdominal discomfort.

Complex Partial Seizures: Loss of consciousness, jerking of the extremities, confusion, involuntary movement of lips, and inability to speak during a seizure.

Tonic-Clonic Seizures: Loss of consciousness for 2 to 5 minutes, rapid and violent jerking movements, tongue biting, shortness of breath, cyanosis, and disruption of breathing may occur.

An aura may appear before seizure activity in some cases.

Diagnostics: Electroencephalography (EEG) to see the electrical activity in the brain, CT brain, and MRI of the brain.

Complications: Status epilepticus, which is continuous seizure activity that can cause airway obstruction and brain damage. This is a medical emergency, and maintaining an open airway is a priority.

Drug Therapy: Antiepileptics such as phenobarbital (Sodium Luminal), phenytoin (Dilantin), valproic acid (Depakote), and levetiracetam (Keppra) are commonly used to treat seizures. Levels of the medication are often checked through lab work to maintain a healthy level of medication in the body. Oxygen therapy may be needed during and after a seizure.

Nursing Care: Patients who present with seizure activity must be placed on seizure precautions and closely monitored. Side rails of the beds must be padded. Patients must be given assistance when walking. Keep emergency airway equipment at the bedside. Maintain a patent airway if patient is having a seizure (Ambu bag, suction, and O_2 must be at bedside). → **Never force anything in the mouth or down the throat during a seizure.** As a nurse, you must document seizure activity, if possible (duration, description of movements, and any triggers). Administer medications as ordered. Maintain hydration and nutrition. Most seizures are 1 to 5 minutes in duration.

Parkinson's Disease

Definition: This is a progressive disease caused by decreasing amounts of circulating dopamine (a primary neurotransmitter responsible for motor movement) due to progressive damage to the nerve cells. An insidious weakening of the muscles is a common occurrence with Parkinson's.

Signs and Symptoms: **Muscle rigidity, tremors, dysphagia, difficulty swallowing, urinary retention, decrease in facial expressions, depression, bradykinesia, drooling, and a shuffling gait.** ←

Diagnostics: Lab work such as monitoring dopamine and acetylcholine levels. There are no definitive tests for Parkinson's.

Complications: Progression and worsening of the symptoms.

Drug Therapy: Anti-parkinsonian medications are used to help balance dopamine and acetylcholine levels. Dopaminergics such as carbidopa/levodopa (Sinemet) and amantadine (Symmetrel) are commonly used. An anticholinergic such as benztropine mesylate (Cogentin) is commonly used.

Nursing Care: **Promote and teach the patient the importance of maintaining a safe environment in view of an increased risk of falls.** ← Offer assistive devices such as a cane or walker. Decrease clutter in the room. Assist with daily activities. Assess the patient's ability to swallow, and increase calorie intake. If the patient is having difficulty swallowing, a soft diet or pureed diet may be ordered. Physical therapy is ordered to maintain muscle strength and range of motion. Educate and provide emotional support to both to patients and their families.

Multiple Sclerosis

Definition: Multiple sclerosis (MS) is an autoimmune and progressive disease caused by the destruction of the myelin tissue in the brain. The destruction of the myelin tissue leads to a progressive loss of function.

Signs and Symptoms: Generalized weakness, muscle pain, tremors, dizziness, numbness, fatigue, diplopia (double vision), decreased concentration, disruption in speech, confusion, muscle spasms, abnormal reflexes, loss of sensory function, urinary retention, and incontinence.

Diagnostics: There are no definitive tests for MS. MRI of the brain or testing of the cerebrospinal fluid may be assessed.

Complications: Progression and worsening of symptoms. If left untreated complete loss of muscle function may occur.

Drug Therapy: **Corticosteroids such as prednisone or IV methylprednisolone (SoluMedrol) are used to treat attacks.** ← Plasmapheresis may be used if corticosteroids are ineffective. Beta-interferons such as Avonex, Betaseron, and Rebif are commonly used. To decrease muscle spasms, muscle relaxers such as baclofen (Lioresal) or diazepam (Valium) are used. Antidepressants may be administered. Pain medications are also used.

Nursing Care: Provide periods of rest to decrease fatigue. Fall precautions may be needed when patients are experiencing periods of weakness. Assistive devices may be needed. Monitor bowel and urinary function, and monitor for urinary retention. In view of the loss of sensory function, teach patients to avoid extreme temperatures. Patients who are on long-term steroids may have thin and fragile skin; hence, use precaution to prevent skin tears. Adequate nutrition and hydration are needed.

Amyotrophic Lateral Sclerosis

Definition: Also known as Lou Gehrig's disease, amyotrophic lateral sclerosis (ALS) causes progressive damage to the nerves that eventually impairs involuntary muscle movements. (The famous "Ice Bucket Challenge" was created to raise money for ALS.)

Signs and Symptoms: Muscle cramping, muscle weakness, twitching, fatigue, and, eventually, loss of all motor function.

Diagnostics: Electromyography and muscle biopsy.

Complications: Complete muscle loss and death.

Drug Therapy: Corticosteroids and riluzole (Rilutek).

Nursing Care: Maintain safety in view of the risk of falls. Assist with daily activities. Assistive devices may be used. Advise patients to conserve energy and ensure periods of rest. Monitor hydration and nutrition. Assist with eating or drinking by placing patients at a 90 degree angle to prevent aspiration. Family and patient teaching is needed, along with emotional support.

Myasthenia Gravis

Definition: This is a progressive autoimmune disorder caused by decreased levels of acetylcholine and damage to the nerve impulses.

Signs and Symptoms: Muscle weakness, diplopia (double vision), ptosis (drooping of the eyelids), difficulty swallowing, loss of bowel and urinary function, impaired breathing, fatigue, and twitching.

→ *Diagnostics:* **Tensilon test (i.e., when IV Tensilon is administered, temporary relief of muscle weakness occurs)**; electromyography is used to evaluate muscle responses to various stimuli; CT or MRI of the brain; lab work to obtain acetylcholine levels.

Complications: Respiratory failure, paralysis, and worsening of symptoms. Two different crises may occur: a cholinergic crisis or a myasthenic crisis. A cholinergic crisis is a toxic side effect of anticholinesterase medication. **Symptoms are nausea, vomiting, diarrhea, decreased BP, muscle spasms, and visual changes.** If this occurs, anticholinesterase medications are held, and the antidote atropine, which should be kept at the bedside, should be administered. Myasthenic crisis occurs when there is muscle weakness and respiratory failure. **Symptoms are shortness of breath, labored breathing, respiratory failure/distress, decrease in O_2 levels, increased BP/HR, and difficulty swallowing.** This is considered a medical emergency, and mechanical ventilation may be needed. Anticholinesterase medications are administered, as well.

Drug Therapy: Anticholinesterase medications such as neostigmine (Prostigmin) and pyridostigmine (Mestinon) are administered. Corticosteroids or plasmapheresis may also be used.

Nursing Care: Proper medication administration is crucial to avoid crises. Use diagnostic tests to determine what type of crisis is occurring. Treat respiratory distress or any changes immediately. Myasthenic crisis is a medical emergency. Maintain airway and oxygen levels. Aspiration precautions are in place. Assist patients with walking, using assistive devices when needed. Adequate rest periods are needed to decrease fatigue. Visual changes such as ptosis and diplopia can become severe, so provide a safe environment. Provide a high-calorie diet with adequate hydration.

Guillain-Barré Syndrome

Definition: This condition involves destruction of the myelin sheath, causing damage to the peripheral nervous system. It can occur rapidly, causing impairment of both the motor and the sensory functions. It most often occurs days or weeks after a respiratory infection.

Signs and Symptoms: Hypotension, bradycardia, weakness, difficulty speaking, difficulty chewing and swallowing, paralysis, and respiratory changes. **Symptoms appear quickly over a course of 1 to 2 days.** If respiratory failure occurs, mechanical ventilation may be needed.

Diagnostics: Lumbar puncture to determine if there is an increase of protein in the cerebrospinal fluid, assessment of symptoms, and electromyography to test muscle response.

Complications: Respiratory distress/failure, long-term paralysis, and death if left untreated.

Drug Therapy: Corticosteroids, immunoglobulin (IVIG), and immunosuppressive medications are often administered. **IVIG is used to replace protein in patients who lack antibodies to help fight infections. Plasmapheresis may also be administered to remove damaged antibodies and replace them with healthy ones to help fight infections.** Antibiotics will also be administered.

Nursing Care: Assess mental status, respiratory status, and any changes in vital signs. Maintain a patent airway. If needed, the patient may be placed on mechanical ventilation. Suction patient as needed. Keep the head of the bed (HOB) at a 45° angle. Assess the patient's ability to swallow, and keep NPO (nothing by mouth) if patient is choking or having difficulty eating. Cardiac monitoring may be ordered for the patient. Pressure relief devices such as pneumatic boots or TED hose are applied to facilitate circulation. Ensure fall precautions are in place, and assist patient with walking and use of assistive devices. Physical therapy will be ordered in the recovery phase. Patient teaching and emotional support is provided. This diagnosis can be difficult for patients owing to the rapid onset and severity of symptoms.

Meningitis

Definition: This is a viral or bacterial infection that causes inflammation of the meninges of the brain and spinal cord. Bacterial meningitis is more severe than viral. Meningococcal meningitis is contagious and transmitted through droplets.

Signs and Symptoms: **Stiff neck, headache,** photophobia, nausea/vomiting, fever, rash, confusion, irritability, positive Kernig and Brudzinski signs.

Diagnostics: Lumbar puncture to test cerebrospinal fluid, elevated WBCs, CT scan, CBC, CMP, and blood cultures.

Complications: Increased intracranial pressure, seizures, paralysis, and if left untreated, brain damage.

Drug Therapy: Corticosteroids, IV antibiotics, anticonvulsants, and oxygen therapy, if needed.

Nursing Care: These patients are placed on droplet precautions until the results of the culture distinguish what type of meningitis is present. Administer medications as ordered. Assess respiratory status, mental status, and vital signs. Assess for complications. Ensure seizure precautions are in place. **If photophobia is present, decreased stimuli and dim lighting may be needed.** Hydration through IVF may be administered. Provide comfort.

Encephalopathy

Definition: This is an infection that causes inflammation of the brain and central nervous system. Encephalopathy can be caused by medications, toxins, **alcohol withdrawal,** substance abuse, and infection. ←

Signs and Symptoms: Changes in mental status, loss of motor function, lethargy, fatigue, profound weakness, personality changes, involuntary movement, tremors, and respiratory changes.

Diagnostics: Lab work, WBC, ammonia testing CSF through a lumbar puncture, and CT of the brain.

Complications: Permanent brain damage.

Drug Therapy: Antibiotics, anticonvulsants, and IV hydration. Treat the underlying cause.

Nursing Care: Assess respiratory and mental status. Provide safety, especially if patients are experiencing confusion. Assist with daily activities. Assess the swallow and gag reflex to determine the patient's ability to swallow without aspirating or choking. Place patient on aspiration precautions. Administer medications as ordered. Treat the underlying cause.

Increased Intracranial Pressure (ICP)

Definition: Increased intracranial pressure is caused by increased fluid in the brain tissue. ICP can be caused by hemorrhage, stroke, trauma, hydrocephalus, tumor, edema, and brain injury.

Signs and Symptoms: Headache, **change in mental status (first sign)**, nausea/vomiting, decreased pulse and increased systolic blood pressure, vision changes, decreased motor function, seizures, changes in speech, respiratory changes, and changes in posture. ←

Diagnostics: Intracranial pressure monitoring, CT scan, MRI, ABGs, and lumbar puncture. Assess neuro status, pupil response, and gait. Use the Glasgow Coma Scale to assess neurological status.

Complications: Seizures and permanent brain damage.

Drug Therapy: **Osmotic diuretics such as mannitol (Osmitrol), corticosteroids, IVF such as D5, anticonvulsants, antihypertensives, and antibiotics to prevent infection.** ←

Surgical Measures: A ventriculoperitoneal shunt may be placed to drain fluid from the brain into the peritoneum.

Preoperative and postoperative teaching is needed. Keep the patient NPO before surgery.

Nursing Care: Patients who are diagnosed with increased intracranial pressure are placed in the ICU for frequent neuro checks and monitoring. Assess mental status, vital signs, and respiratory status. Monitor the ICP; normal range is 5 to 15 mmHg. Mechanical ventilation may be needed to enhance oxygen intake. **Keep head and neck midline, and keep the HOB at a 45° angle. Avoid any sudden changes in movement.** Also avoid hip flexion. Initiate seizure precautions. A Foley catheter may be placed. Administer medications as ordered. Monitor vital signs, I/Os, and changes in mental status. Fluid restriction may be ordered. The patient is placed on strict bed rest. If the patient is unconscious, maintain skin integrity, tube feedings, mouth care, and perianal care.

Spinal Cord Injury

Definition: This is caused by trauma or damage to the spinal cord. Spinal cord injury can be thoracic, lumbar, or cervical. Symptoms and severity can vary based on the level of injury. Injuries to C4 and above cause respiratory impairment, necessitating ventilation. An injury at the C1 to C8 level causes paralysis of all four extremities. An injury at the C6 to C8 level causes lower extremity paralysis with movement in the upper extremities. An injury that occurs at the T1 to T4 level has lower extremity paralysis, with ability to move upper extremities. Several complications can occur with spinal cord injury depending on the location of trauma to the spine.

Types of Injuries: **Central cord syndrome, anterior cord syndrome, posterior cord syndrome, conus medullaris syndrome, and Brown-Séquard syndrome. The two most commonly tested are the conus medullaris syndrome and Brown-Séquard syndrome.**

Signs and Symptoms:

Severity of symptoms is measured by on the level of damage and location of the injury. Injuries at C3 to C5 will cause respiratory failure, and patients need to be placed on mechanical ventilation immediately. Patients with injuries at C6 or higher will experience severe hypertension, loss of bladder function, neurogenic bladder, lack of sensation, hypertension, and loss of motor function. Patients with injuries at T6 and above can develop autonomic dysreflexia, severe hypertension, and decreased pulse.

General symptoms are hypertension, urinary retention, skin ulcers, paralytic ileus, weight loss, deep vein thrombosis, pulmonary embolism, immobility, and pain.

Diagnostics: CT scan, MRI of the brain, EKG, electrolytes, ABGs, and neurological symptoms that may be present.

Complications: Many complications can arise from spinal cord injury; two of the main complications are (a) autonomic dysreflexia and (b) spinal cord shock. Autonomic dysreflexia occurs with injuries at T6 and higher. It can be life threatening and needs to be treated immediately. Symptoms are distended (full) bladder, blurred vision, headache, hypertension, sweating, and bradycardia. **Treatment is elevating the HOB to 45°, loosening clothing, and checking the Foley catheter for kinks that can possibly cause the bladder to be full. Assess the bladder/bowel, monitor output, assessing BP every 15 minutes, administering hypertensive medications, and notify the physician immediately.** ←

Spinal cord shock is caused by absence of reflexes, which usually occurs a few hours after the injury and can last for several months. Autonomic dysreflexia can result from spinal cord shock. **Signs and symptoms are paralysis, hypotension, bradycardia, loss of reflexes, profuse sweating, and EKG changes.** ← Treatment includes monitoring and controlling hypotension and bradycardia, and frequent monitoring of vital signs. Reflexes have to be assessed frequently.

Drug Therapy: Treatment of bradycardia is IV fluids, corticosteroids (IV solumedrol), pain medications, and vasopressors to increase vasodilation. Diuretics such as furosemide (Lasix) are used to increase diuresis and decrease edema. Anticoagulants such as enoxaparin (Lovenox) are used to prevent blood clots. Pain medications may be used for comfort, stool softeners such as Colace or Senna may also be prescribed, as well as anticonvulsants to prevent seizures. Provide the patient with emotional comfort.

Nursing Care: Assess respiratory status and maintain a patent airway; the patient may need to be placed on mechanical ventilation. Assess for infection, ABGs, vital signs, intake, and output. Cardiac monitoring is ordered. TED hose and pneumatic boots are applied to decrease the risk of clots. To increase BP and pulse, intravenous fluids and vasopressors are administered. Patients' skin integrity needs to be maintained by turning and repositioning, using an air mattress, and applying barrier cream. **To avoid complications, monitor bowel and bladder function. Maintain a patent Foley catheter, assess for abdominal distension, assess for bowel sounds, and administer stool softeners.** ← A nasogastric tube

(NGT) may need to be placed if a bowel obstruction occurs. Remember to keep the head and neck aligned at all times with no hip flexion. Traction such as a halo may be used to maintain alignment. Assess for other complications such as pneumonia, which can result from lack of mobility. Assess neurological status every hour, and call physician with any changes.

Subarachnoid Hemorrhage/Aneurysm

Definition: A subarachnoid hemorrhage is a collection of blood in the subarachnoid space, typically caused by an aneurysm, which can result in death. An aneurysm is a bleed in the subarachnoid space.

Signs and Symptoms: Mental status changes, headache, nausea, vomiting, increased intracranial pressure, nuchal rigidity, seizures, photophobia, and restlessness.

Diagnostics: CT of the brain, MRI, ABGs, PT/INR, PTT, CBC, and ICP pressure.

Complications: Seizures and death if left untreated.

Drug Therapy: Osmotic diuretics, anticonvulsants, corticosteroids, CCBs, analgesics, oxygen therapy, antipyretics, stool softeners, and aminocaproic acid (Amicar).

Nursing Care: Assess respiratory status and maintain patent airway. Keep patient neck and head aligned to prevent further damage and increase ICP. Closely monitor neurological status. Tell patients to avoid factors that can increase pressure such as blowing the nose, heavy lifting, and bending. CSF can leak from the nose and ears; assess both frequently. Administer medications as ordered. Surgery such as a craniotomy may be needed. Continue to monitor for complications.

ENDOCRINE DISORDERS

Assessing a Patient With Endocrine Disorders

Review the endocrine system in your anatomy and physiology book. Obtain a health history from the patient, assessing for any chronic or new symptoms. There are many complex disorders that involve the endocrine system. I will go over each disorder and highlight the most frequently tested information.

Endocrine Diagnostics

Labs: Amylase, lipase, thyroxine (T4), triiodothyronine (T3), thyroid-stimulating hormone (TSH), Hgb A1C, BUN/Cr, serum glucose, fasting glucose, growth hormone, and various urine tests. Normal values are as follows:

- Urine specific gravity: 1.003 to 1.030
- Blood glucose: 70 to 110 mg/dL
- Hgb A1C: 4% to 6%
- Lipase: 10 to 160 U/L
- Amylase serum: 40 to 140 U/L
- T4: 5 to 12 mcg/dL
- TSH: 0.4 to 4.2 mIU/L

CT scan or ultrasound of the thyroid and adrenal glands may be done.

Disorders of the Pituitary: Diabetes Insipidus (DI) and Syndrome of Inappropriate Antidiuretic Hormone (SIADH)

Definition: Diabetes insipidus is a decrease in the level of antidiuretic hormone (ADH) with a resulting increase in urine osmolarity. Kidney function is impaired owing to the lack of ADH, leading to excessive water loss and concentraton of urine. SIADH is the continuous release of or increase in ADH. **Head injury, trauma, and stroke can all cause alterations in ADH levels.** ←

Signs and Symptoms: **3Ps—polydipsia (excessive thirst), polyuria (frequent urination), and polyphagia (frequent hunger). Other symptoms include decreased urine specific gravity, hypernatremia, weight loss, nausea, decreased BP, muscle pain, and fatigue. Signs and symptoms of SIADH are low urine output, fatigue, increased urine specific gravity, weight loss, hyponatremia, and edema.** ←

Diagnostics: ADH levels, urine specific gravity, urine osmolarity, electrolytes, and clinical symptoms.

Complications: Worsening of symptoms, seizure with SIADH, and shock.

Drug Therapy: DI is treated with ADH replacement medications such as desmopressin (DDAVP) by the intranasal route and vasopressin (Pitressin) as first-line treatment. Treatment for SIADH is a diuretic such as furosemide (Lasix); sodium may be administered; declomycin (Demeclocycline) or lithium carbonate (Lithobid) is used to block ADH production and increase urine production.

Nursing Care: Assess patient vital signs, intake, and output. Daily weights are important to assess for urinary retention.

Strict intake and output must be recorded. Monitor labs. Fluid restriction may be needed for patients with SIADH. Assess mental status for any changes.

Adrenal Disorders: Cushing's Syndrome and Addison's Disease

Cushing's Syndrome

Definition: This condition is caused by an increase in adrenal hormones such as adrenocorticotropic hormone (ACTH), glucocorticoids, and cortisol. It can be caused by pituitary tumor or steroid use.

Signs and Symptoms: Weight gain, moon face, dry skin, buffalo hump, hypokalemia, increased glucose levels, purple striae, hypertension, muscle wasting, poor healing, truncal obesity, osteoporosis, and bruising.

Diagnostics: Lab work such as cortisol, ACTH levels, glucose, and electrolytes. CT and MRI of the pituitary gland.

Complications: Hypertension, CHF, and worsening of symptoms.

→ *Drug Therapy:* Potassium may be administered. **Corticosteroids may be ordered to help relieve symptoms.**

Nursing Care: Treat the underlying cause. Surgical removal of the tumor or adrenalectomy may be necessary. Monitor hormone levels and electrolytes. Monitor blood glucose and ACTH levels. Administer steroids as ordered. Steroids also increase glucose levels; it is important to monitor and treat as ordered. Monitor for any complications.

Addison's Disease

Definition: This is an autoimmune disorder caused by a decrease in mineralocorticoids (which control Na and K levels) and glucocorticoids. It can occur after an adrenalectomy.

Signs and Symptoms: Fatigue, weakness, weight loss, hypotension, hyperkalemia, hyponatremia, nausea, vomiting, and diarrhea.

Diagnostics: Labs such as glucose levels, cortisol levels, ACTH, electrolytes, and presentation of symptoms. ACTH stimulation tests.

Complications: Addison's crisis may occur and can lead to death if left untreated. It can be caused by high levels of stress or high levels of steroids. Signs and symptoms are hypotension, increased heart rate, peak T waves, decreased sodium, increased potassium, dehydration, and cyanosis. Shock can occur if left untreated. It is treated with glucocorticoids such as hydrocortisone sodium succinate (Solu-Cortef) to replace hormones; calcium with vitamin D to increase calcium levels; and intravenous fluids. Monitor glucose and BP levels closely.

Drug Therapy: Corticosteroids therapy such as hydrocortisone, sodium, fluids, and dextrose. **Here is a little trick: "Addison's" means to *add* steroids for treatment.** ←

Nursing Care: Monitor vital signs (especially BP), glucose levels, and signs of Addison's disease. Evaluate for edema and urinary retention. Check daily weight. Maintain a low-stress environment. Minimize the risk of infection. Patients must be placed on a high-protein, low-potassium diet. Patients are placed on bed rest to conserve energy.

Hypothyroidism and Hyperthyroidism

Hypothyroidism

Definition: This is a condition in which there is a decrease in thyroid hormones T3 and T4 and an increase in TSH levels.

Signs and Symptoms: Fatigue, weakness, slowed speech, weight gain, dry skin, brittle nails, cold intolerance, constipation, bradycardia, decreased activity, myxedema (swelling of face/eyes). Cardiac changes may be present, and a goiter (growth on the thyroid) can cause hypothyroidism.

Diagnostics: Thyroid levels, glucose levels, and a CT scan of the thyroid to assess for a goiter.

Complications: Hypothyroidism can lead to *myxedema coma*, characterized by a decrease in heart rate, low sodium, and low blood sugar. Patients may present with respiratory difficulty. This is a medical emergency, and the physician must be notified immediately. Administration of fluids, corticosteroids, levothyroxine (Synthroid), and glucose can decrease the severity of complications. Monitor vital signs and labs. **Don't forget your ABCs!** ←

Drug Therapy: Thyroid replacement such as levothyroxine (Synthroid).

Nursing Care: The focus of care is proper administration of medication and patient education. Monitor thyroid levels. Monitor electrolytes. Keep the patient's environment stress-free and warm. Supply the patient with extra blankets to help with intolerance to cold. Teach patients the signs and symptoms of hyperthyroidism and myxedema coma.

Hyperthyroidism (Graves' Disease)

Definition: This is an autoimmune disorder that causes an increase in T3 and T4 thyroid hormones. A decrease in iodine and TSH is seen. It is typically caused by a goiter.

Signs and Symptoms: Hypertension, increased heart rate, weight loss, heat intolerance, exophthalmos (protruding eyeballs), hair loss, tremors, and cardiac arrhythmias.

Diagnostics: Increased T3 and T4 levels. Decrease in TSH levels. Obtain iodine levels.

Complications: Thyroid storm or thyrotoxic crisis can occur. Signs and symptoms are severely increased, and include hyperpyrexia, nausea, vomiting, diarrhea, and increased heart rate and blood pressure. Cardiac arrhythmias are seen on the EKG. Treatment includes administering oxygen, treating arrhythmias, administering antithyroid medications, iodine, beta-blockers, acetaminophen (Tylenol), and steroids. A thyroidectomy may be needed.

Surgical Measures: A thyroidectomy may be needed to treat hyperthyroidism. Preoperative and postoperative teachings are needed. → **Monitor for complications such as thyroid storm and hypothyroidism. After surgery, it is important to keep a trach kit at the bedside, because respiratory complications can occur.** Assess labs such as electrolytes, glucose, and calcium levels. A thyroidectomy can cause low calcium levels. Assess for Chvostek's and Trousseau's signs.

Drug Therapy: The purpose of drug therapy is to maintain thyroid levels at a therapeutic level. Antithyroid medications include methimazole (Tapazole) or Lugol's solution. Lugol's solution can stain teeth and should be given orally with a straw. To control heart rate, beta-adrenergic blockers such as atenolol (Tenormin) are used.

Nursing Care: Graves' disease is treated with medications and patient education on monitoring for complications. Monitor vital signs and electrolytes. Maintain a high-protein diet to treat weight loss. Maintain a cool environment. The patient may be placed on a cardiac monitor to assess for cardiac arrhythmias. Continue to monitor thyroid levels. Assess and treat complications if they arise. Monitor and maintain airway if respiratory distress occurs.

Hyperparathyroidism and Hypoparathyroidism

Hyperparathyroidism

Definition: This is caused by increased secretion of parathyroid hormone (PTH) from the parathyroid gland. **The parathyroid gland controls calcium and phosphorus levels.** When there is an increase in PTH levels, calcium is increased and phosphorus is decreased. Hyperparathyroidism can be caused by a tumor on the parathyroid gland.

Signs and Symptoms: **Hypercalcemia, hypophosphatemia, increase in blood pressure, muscle pain, constipation, cardiac dysrhythmias, broken bones, kidney stones, nausea, vomiting, and irritability.**

Diagnostics: Increased PTH levels, decreased phosphorus, increased calcium, CT scan, bone density, and x-rays.

Complications: Bone damage and kidney damage.

Drug Therapy: Administer medications such as cinacalet (Sensipar) to increase calcium in the blood. Administer loop diuretics to excrete calcium levels. Biophosphonates are also used to treat osteoporosis and prevent the loss of calcium from the bones.

Surgical Measures: **A parathyroidectomy may be needed.** Preoperative and postoperative teaching is needed. **IV calcium is given to prevent postoperative hypocalcemia.** Assess for respiratory distress, incision, and drainage from the surgical site, and notify the physician of any complications.

Nursing Care: Administer medications as ordered. Monitor calcium intake. Administer intravenous fluids. Fall risk precautions should be in place due to an increased risk of bone fractures. Assistive devices are used to promote a steady gait. Cardiac monitoring may be ordered. Monitor vital signs. Assess for kidney stones.

Hypoparathyroidism

Definition: In this condition, there is a decrease in PTH levels, an increase in phosphorus, and a decrease in calcium levels. Hypoparathyroidism can be caused by parathyroidectomy, which is the surgical removal of the parathyroid gland.

Signs and Symptoms: Hypocalcemia, hyperphosphatemia, tetany, **positive Chvostek's and Trousseau's signs, cardiac dysrhythmias, hair loss, abdominal cramping, nausea, vomiting, and laryngospasms. Chvostek's sign is present when the facial nerve is stimulated and eye twitching occurs. Trousseau's sign is present when a blood pressure cuff is applied to the arm and spasms occur in the upper extremity.** Laryngospasms can be fatal and cause respiratory failure.

Diagnostics: Parathyroid levels, x-ray of the glands, electrolytes, calcium, and phosphorus levels.

Complications: Respiratory distress and seizures.

Drug Therapy: Administration of IV calcium, calcium supplements, and vitamin D.

Nursing Care: Administer medications as ordered. Monitor calcium and phosphorus levels. Maintain seizure precautions. Keep a trach kit at the patient's bedside in case respiratory distress occurs. Maintain an open airway, and assess for signs of respiratory distress.

Diabetes Mellitus (DM)

Definition: This is a pancreatic disorder caused by decreased or inadequate insulin production. The beta cells in the islets of Langerhans secrete insulin, which is used to control glucose levels in the body. There are two types of diabetes mellitus: Type 1 and type 2. In type 1, also known as *insulin-dependent diabetes mellitus,* beta cells of the pancreas do not produce enough of the hormone insulin. Type 1 is usually diagnosed in childhood. It is important to assess and avoid ketoacidosis in patients with type 1 DM. In type 2, known as *non–insulin-dependent diabetes mellitus,* the body develops resistance to insulin production. Type 2 is most commonly seen in adults, and often occurs as a result of lifestyle factors (e.g., obesity).

Signs and Symptoms: The 3Ps are the first signs of DM: polydipsia, polyuria, and polyphagia. Patients with type 1 have symptoms of 3Ps, fatigue, weight loss, and blurred vision, and symptoms occur rapidly. Those with type 2 have symptoms of 3Ps, weight gain, fatigue, increase in infections, and blurred vision, and can be asymptomatic. Type 2 can be asymptomatic for years and develop over a long period of time.

→ *Diagnostics:* **Serum glucose levels (normal range is 60 to 100 mg/dL, fasting blood glucose, Hgb A1C (4% to 6%), BUN/Cr, and urine tests (looking for ketones).**

Complications: Among the many complications of DM, are those listed below:

- *Diabetic Ketoacidosis (DKA):* This occurs in DM type 1, when the body responds to its inability to use glucose for fuel by breaking down proteins into ketones that accumulate in the bloodstream. Symptoms include glucose levels of 300 to 800 mg/dL, metabolic acidosis, ketones in the urine, fruity breath, weakness, alteration in K levels, and dehydration. DKA needs to be treated immediately, with an insulin drip, and fluids are needed.

- *Hyperglycemic Hyperosmolar Nonketotic Syndrome (HHS):* This occurs in patients with DM type 2. It causes severe dehydration with a marked increase in glucose levels (glucose levels of above 600 mg/dL). Symptoms are extreme thirst, weakness, confusion, loss of vision, and fever. Treatment includes insulin and intravenous fluids.
- *Hypoglycemia:* This occurs when the blood sugar levels go below 70 mg/dL. It can occur as a side effect of insulin. Symptoms are dizziness, visual changes, mental status changes, sweating, tachycardia, nervousness, numbness, syncope, and fatigue. Treatment is to increase blood glucose levels. Orange juice (6 ounces) and graham crackers can be given, then blood glucose level should be rechecked in 15 minutes. If blood glucose remains low, intravenous D5 must be administered to increase glucose levels. Continue to assess blood glucose.
- *Diabetic Nephropathy:* This is progressive damage to the kidneys as a result of end-stage renal disease caused by uncontrolled DM.
- *Diabetic Neuropathy:* Neuropathy in DM occurs when there is a lack of blood supply to the nerves, and causes pain, numbness, and tingling in the feet and fingertips. Patients with DM should be referred to a podiatrist. Due to the lack of feeling in their feet, patients are at risk for infections and wounds. *Diabetic ulcers* often occur from wounds or infection in the feet.

Drug Therapy:

Oral hypoglycemic medications:

- Sulfonylureas such as glimepiride (Amaryl) or glipizide (Glucotrol).
- Biguanides such as metformin (Glucophage).
- Alpha-glucosidase inhibitors such as acarbose (Precose) or miglitol (Glyset).
- Thiazolidinedione such as pioglitazone (Actos) or rosiglitazone (Avandia).
- Meglitinides such as nateglinide (Starlix) or repaglinide (Prandin).
- Dipeptidyl peptidase-4 such as stigliptin (Januvia).

Oral hypoglycemic medications are discussed in Chapter 5 in greater detail. This is just to give you an idea of the various types of medications given. Typically, patients take these medications twice a day, in the morning and evening.

Insulin:

- Rapid-acting insulin has an onset of 15 minutes, peaks in 60 to 90 minutes, and lasts 3 to 4 hours. Types are lispro (Humalog) and aspart.
- Short-acting insulin has an onset of 30 minutes to 1 hour, peaks in 2 to 3 hours, and lasts 3 to 6 hours. Regular insulin is short-acting insulin.
- Intermediate insulin has an onset of 2 to 4 hours, peaks in 4 to 10 hours, and lasts for 10 to 16 hours. One type of intermediate insulin is NPH. It can be mixed with regular insulin.
- Long-acting insulin has an onset of 1 to 2 hours, no peak, and lasts for 24 hours. Types are glargine (Lantus) and detemir (Levemir).

Insulin is discussed in more detail in Chapter 5. Rapid-acting and short-acting insulin is administered at mealtimes and bedtime with glucose levels checked before administration. An insulin sliding scale is used to determine how much insulin is to be given based on the patient's glucose level. Insulin must be refrigerated and the expiration date (expires in 30 days from opening) checked before administering. Insulin is given subcutaneously and sites should be rotated at each injection. Always wash hands and use an alcohol wipe to clean the skin before injecting. If the patient is hypoglycemic or blood glucose is below 70 mg/dL, insulin should be held, and orange juice or D5 should be given. → **When mixing NPH and regular insulin, remember to always mix the clear insulin first, which is regular insulin, and then the NPH, which is cloudy. Clear before cloudy.**

Nursing Care: DM can often be treated with diet, exercise, and medications. Patient education is needed to provide information about the disease and promote a healthy lifestyle, as well as to avoid complications that could arise if DM is left untreated. The importance of an exercise regimen and weight control is emphasized. A diabetic diet includes an intake of 1,800 to 2,000 daily calories and excludes food with sugars to maintain healthy glucose levels. Blood glucose levels should always be checked before insulin administration, with the use of a sliding scale. Always monitor for signs of hypoglycemia. Patients with diabetes are also susceptible to infections and wounds. A podiatrist should be seen monthly. Other medications such as beta-adrenergic blockers, including metoprolol (Lopressor) and atenolol (Tenormin), can mask symptoms of hypoglycemia, and corticosteroids can increase blood glucose levels.

GASTROINTESTINAL DISORDERS (GI)

Assessing a Patient With Gastrointestinal Disorders

Review the gastrointestinal system in your anatomy and physiology book. Obtain a health history from the patient, assessing for any chronic or new symptoms. Conduct an abdominal exam, listening for bowel sounds, palpating the abdomen, assessing for pain, and assessing for constipation, nausea, or vomiting.

Gastrointestinal Diagnostics

Lab Work: WBCs, CBC, CMP, liver enzymes, hemoglobin, hematocrit, BUN/Cr, liver function tests, amylase, and lipase.

Abdominal X-ray/Kidney, Ureter, and Bladder (KUB): This is used to obtain images of the abdomen.

Endoscopy: This is the insertion of a scope to view the upper GI tract.

Colonoscopy: This is the insertion of a scope to view the lower GI tract.

Sigmoidoscopy: This is the insertion of a scope in the sigmoid colon.

Abdominal CT Scan or Ultrasound: This produces images of the abdomen.

Barium Studies: Barium is swallowed and highlights the abdomen using an x-ray.

Stool Culture: Stool is tested for blood and other pathogens.

Gastroesophageal Reflux Disease (GERD)

Definition: In GERD, **a decrease in function of the pyloric sphincter causes the gastric contents to push back into the esophagus, leading to heartburn and discomfort.** For those who suffer from GERD, lay off the tacos and spicy foods! ←

Signs and Symptoms: Pain and burning sensation in the chest and stomach, difficulty swallowing, pain after eating, nausea and vomiting.

Diagnostics: pH levels, esophagoscopy, and presentation of symptoms.

Complications: Aspiration pneumonia and dental erosion from the gastric acid.

Drug Therapy: Histamine H_2 receptor antagonists such as ranitidine (Zantac), cimetidine (Tagamet), and famotidine (Pepcid); proton pump inhibitors such as omeprazole

(Prilosec) and pantoprazole (Protonix); and antacids such as TUMS or Maalox are commonly prescribed. The surgical procedure fundoplication can be performed to decrease reflux.

Nursing Care: To prevent GERD, patients should maintain a bland diet. Spicy and fatty foods, caffeine, and sodas can → increase symptoms. **Patients are instructed to take an antacid before eating and remain sitting up for an hour after eating.** Avoid drinking 2 hours before bedtime. Administer medication as ordered.

Ulcerative Colitis

Definition: This is an inflammation of the bowel and digestive tract.

Signs and Symptoms: Abdominal pain, bloody stool, severe diarrhea, weight loss, loss of electrolytes, and dehydration.

Diagnostics: Stool sample, CT of the abdomen, colonoscopy, and WBC for infection.

Complications: Perforated bowel or severe dehydration.

Drug Therapy: Antibiotics, probiotics, immunosuppressants, analgesics, antidiarrheals, anti-inflammatories, and corticosteroids to decrease inflammation.

Surgical Measures: Protocolectomy, ileostomy, and colostomy may be needed if symptoms become severe or chronic.

Nursing Care: Assess labs and stool, and monitor for bloody stools. Administer medications as ordered. Intravenous fluids may be administered. Patients should maintain a low-fiber diet, while trying to avoid alcohol, caffeine, and spicy foods. Stress can worsen ulcerative colitis. If surgery is needed, preoperative and postoperative teaching is necessary.

Crohn's Disease

Definition: This is a chronic inflammation of the GI system and a type of inflammatory bowel disease.

Signs and Symptoms: Diarrhea, abdominal pain, fatigue, mouth sores, weight loss, and fever.

Diagnostics: MRI or CT of the abdomen, colonoscopy, small bowel series, capsule endoscopy, sigmoidoscopy, and lab work for bleeding and infection.

Complications: Severe dehydration and worsening of symptoms.

Drug Therapy: Oral 5-aminosalicylates such as sulfasalazine (Azulfidine) and mesalamine (Pentasa). Corticosteroids are used to decrease inflammation. Immunosuppressant medications, antidiarrheals, antibiotics, and nutritional supplements are ordered.

Nursing Care: Monitor hydration status and correct fluid and electrolyte losses due to diarrhea. A high-calorie diet is needed to treat weight loss. Administer medications as ordered. Flare-ups can occur, which can be painful and severe. Monitor bowel for bloody stools. Intravenous fluids may be administered.

Diverticulitis/Diverticulosis

Definition: Diverticulitis is an inflammation of sac-like herniations in the bowel lining. Diverticulosis is the condition of having diverticuli.

Signs and Symptoms: Abdominal pain, abdominal distension, nausea, vomiting, fever, tarry stools, and constipation.

Diagnostics: CT or ultrasound of the abdomen, barium enema, and lab work (WBCs/CRP).

Complications: Perforated or obstructed bowel.

Drug Therapy: Antibiotics, analgesics, IV fluids, pain medications, and anticholinergics.

Nursing Care: Keep patient NPO until symptoms resolve. **Patients with diverticulitis should avoid eating foods with seeds such as strawberries or sesame seeds.** ← Administer medications as ordered. Surgery may be needed if a complication arises.

Gastroenteritis

Definition: This is an inflammation of the stomach and small bowel. It can be caused by *E. coli* or staph infection.

Signs and Symptoms: Abdominal cramping, abdominal distension, nausea, vomiting, diarrhea, weight loss, and fever.

Diagnostics: Stool culture and CT of the abdomen.

Complications: Worsening of the symptoms.

Drug Therapy: Antibiotics, antiemetics, pain medication, and intravenous fluids.

Nursing Care: Administer medications as ordered. Keep patient NPO until symptoms resolve. Obtain bowel specimens.

Clostridium difficile (C. diff)

Definition: A bacterial infection caused by the organism *C. difficile*, which attacks the intestines.

Signs and Symptoms: Severe diarrhea, watery stool, foul-smelling stool, fever, weight loss, dehydration, and pain.

Diagnostics: Stool sample and culture, WBCs, and monitoring electrolytes.

Complications: Severe dehydration and worsening of infection.

Drug Therapy: IV antibiotics such as metronidazole (Flagyl) or vancomycin are used. A peripherally inserted central catheter (PICC) or midline catheter may need to be placed if vancomycin will be administered. Probiotics should be given as well.

→ *Nursing Care:* **These patients are placed on contact precautions! *C. diff* is contagious and is transmitted through contact. Wash hands with soap and water; hand sanitizer does not remove the *C. diff* organism from the hands.** Wear a gown and gloves when treating these patients. Administer antibiotics as ordered.

Small Bowel Obstruction

Definition: This is an obstruction in the duodenum or jejunum. Small bowel obstruction can be caused by a hernia, volvulus, adhesions, tumors, and ileus.

Signs and Symptoms: Severe nausea and vomiting (bilious emesis), fever, hypoactive bowel sounds, constipation, abdominal distension, and abdominal pain.

→ *Diagnostics:* **CT of the abdomen, KUB, and small bowel series.**

Complications: Sepsis, perforation of the bowel, and aspiration pneumonia.

Drug Therapy: Aggressive antibiotics such as IV Cipro or Flagyl. Antiemetics, analgesics, and pain medications.

→ *Nursing Care:* **If severe nausea or vomiting is persistent, an NGT may be placed to decompress the bowels.** Administer medications as ordered. Assess for aspiration pneumonia. The head of the bed (HOB) should be kept at a 30° to 45° angle. Keep patients NPO until symptoms resolve. Administer intravenous fluids. Assess for dehydration. Surgical measures such as a bowel resection may be needed. Preoperative and postoperative teaching is needed.

Peptic Ulcer Disease

Definition: In this condition, gastric secretions cause erosion of the GI tract, resulting in ulcerations. There are two types of ulcers: (a) gastric and (b) duodenal. **Causes include stress, NSAIDs, alcohol abuse, gastritis, and the bacteria *H. pylori.***

Signs and Symptoms:

Gastric ulcers present with symptoms of left midepigastric pain that radiates to the back and upper abdomen 1 to 2 hours after eating. Other symptoms include nausea, vomiting, weight loss, and burning sensation.

Duodenal ulcers present with symptoms of midepigastric pain that occurs 2 to 4 hours after eating and is relieved when antacids are taken. Other symptoms include burning, cramping, nausea, and vomiting.

Diagnostics: Stool culture, barium studies, abdominal x-ray, esophagogastroduodenoscopy (EGD), and colonoscopy.

Complications: Perforation, obstruction, and hemorrhage.

Drug Therapy: Antibiotics, antacids, H_2 antagonists, proton pump inhibitors, anticholinergics, and cytoprotective agents.

Surgical Measures: Partial gastrectomy, gastric resection, vagotomy, or pyloroplasty may be performed to decrease acid production in the abdomen. A complication that can arise from gastrectomy is *dumping syndrome*. In this syndrome, there is fluid accumulation in the intestine. Symptoms are weakness, epigastric fullness, and cramping, and it occurs right after eating. Prevention involves avoiding large meals and fatty foods.

Nursing Care: **Patients with peptic ulcer disease are encouraged to eat a bland diet.** They should avoid foods that are fatty or spicy, and caffeinated beverages. Smoking cessation is advised. Administer medications as ordered. Use of antacids after eating may help relieve symptoms. An NGT and IVF may be administered to decompress the bowel and treat nausea/vomiting. **Never clamp an NGT without a physician order. Placement of the NGT should be checked at every shift.** Monitor output from the NGT. Surgery may be needed, and patient preoperative and postoperative teaching is needed.

Appendicitis

Definition: Appendicitis is inflammation or obstruction of the appendix.

→ *Signs and Symptoms:* **Abdominal cramping, nausea, vomiting, fever, positive McBurney's sign (right lower quadrant pain) and Rovsing sign (right lower quadrant pain that worsens when the other quadrants are palpated), rebound tenderness, and weight loss.**

Diagnostics: Presentation of symptoms, abdominal x-ray and ultrasound, and lab work (increased WBCs).

Complications: Ruptured appendix, peritonitis, hemorrhage, perforation, and sepsis.

Drug Therapy: Antibiotics, intravenous fluids, and pain medications.

Surgical Measures: Appendectomy and exploratory laparoscopy to diagnose appendicitis.

Nursing Care: Prepare patient for surgery. Administer medications as ordered, and keep patient NPO until surgery occurs. → Try to promote bed rest to decrease pain level. **Never apply heat to the abdomen; apply ice for comfort.** Sudden relief or pain can mean that the appendix has ruptured. It is important to diagnose appendicitis before administering pain medication. Postoperatively, patients remain NPO, and IV fluids are administered. Dressing changes are needed. Patients may have a Jackson-Pratt (JP) drain at the incision site to drain excess fluid. Assess the incision, and drain every 4 hours. Monitor intake and output. Diet should be resumed slowly postoperatively. Assess for infection.

Cholecystitis

Definition: Cholecystitis is inflammation of the gallbladder, which can be caused by gallstones.

Signs and Symptoms: Bloating, nausea/vomiting, pain that occurs 2 to 4 hours after eating, increased heart rate, fever, clay-colored stools, positive Murphy's sign, and fever.

Diagnostics: Abdominal CT scan, ultrasound of the abdomen, hepatobiliary iminodiacetic acid (HIDA) scan, and lab work (elevated WBCs).

Complications: Perforation of the gallbladder and sepsis.

Drug Therapy: Antibiotics, antiemetics, analgesics, and intravenous fluids.

Surgical Measures: A cholecystectomy (removal of the gallbladder) may need to be performed. An NGT may be ordered.

Nursing Care: Patients with cholecystitis may remain NPO until surgery. An NGT may be inserted until surgery. IVF are administered for hydration. Administer pain medication and antibiotics as ordered. Preoperative and postoperative teaching is needed.

Pancreatitis

Definition: Inflammation of the pancreas, which can be caused by alcohol abuse, gallstones, or infection.

Signs and Symptoms: Abdominal pain in the left lower quadrant, dyspnea, nausea, vomiting, tachycardia, jaundice (skin/sclera), positive Cullen's sign (discoloration of the abdomen), positive Turner's sign (blue spotting on flank), weakness, abdominal distension, and fatigue.

Diagnostics: Lab work including pancreatic enzymes, MRI of the abdomen, CT of the abdomen, and urine tests.

Complications: Sepsis.

Drug Therapy: Antibiotics, H_2 antagonists, anticholinergics, and pain medications.

Nursing Care: Patient may be kept NPO until symptoms resolve. IVF and nutritional support may be needed. Smoking and alcohol cessation may be needed. Assess for symptoms of infection. Administer medications as ordered.

Liver Cirrhosis

Definition: This is necrosis and degeneration of the liver commonly caused by alcohol abuse.

Signs and Symptoms: **Jaundice (skin/sclera), anemia, weight loss, fever, peripheral edema, shallow respirations, ascites, abdominal distension, nausea, vomiting, shortness of breath, fatigue, electrolyte imbalance, increased ammonia levels, decreased potassium levels, cardiac changes, asterixis (tremor of the hands), and *fetor hepaticus* (fruity odor on the breath).** ←

Diagnostics: Ultrasound of the abdomen, liver function tests, bilirubin levels, and biopsy of the liver.

Complications: Portal hypertension, encephalopathy, peripheral edema, renal failure, seizures, coma, or death if left untreated.

Drug Therapy: Diuretics, antibiotics, pain medications, lactulose (to promote bowel movements, which decrease ammonia levels), vasopressin, albumin, and enteral nutrition.

Nursing Care: Daily weights and strict intake and output monitoring are needed. Maintain a low-sodium/low-protein diet.

Fluid restriction is ordered. Treat edema and ascites. Provide comfort with pain medication and positioning. Bed rest is required to conserve energy. Alcohol cessation is needed. Monitor signs of withdrawal, and medicate as needed. Measure abdominal girth. Monitor stool output for patients receiving lactulose. Monitor for complications. A paracentesis (drainage of abdominal fluid through needle aspiration) may be performed to treat ascites.

Hepatitis

Definition: Hepatitis is the inflammation of the liver, which can be caused by liver necrosis, viruses, and bacteria. There are several types of hepatitis (A-G). The most common types are hepatitis A, B, and C.

Types of Hepatitis:

Hepatitis A is transmitted through the fecal–oral route and contaminated foods.

Hepatitis B is transmitted through IV needles, sexual activities, bodily fluids, and blood products.

Hepatitis C is transmitted through IV needles and from mother to child.

Signs and Symptoms: Jaundice, fever, weight loss, abdominal cramping, and fatigue. Symptoms occur in stages—preicteric, icteric, and posticteric.

Diagnostics: Lab work such as hepatitis panel, LFTs, and CBC.

Drug Therapy: Antiviral medications and lactulose.

Nursing Care: Diagnostics are used to determine the type of hepatitis. Avoid giving Tylenol to patients who have hepatitis. Monitor for liver failure and other complications. Administer medications as ordered. Monitor liver function tests. A low-fat/high-carbohydrate diet is needed.

Types of Ostomies

An ostomy is a surgical procedure in which the bowel is diverted to an opening in the abdomen so that fecal matter is released through a stoma.

Types of common colostomies:

Colostomy: Opening of the colon through the abdominal wall through a stoma. When assessing the stoma, it should appear pink/red and moist. Stool is released through the stoma, and a colostomy bag is placed to collect the stool.

Ileostomy: Opening of the ileum to the abdominal wall, where stool is drained through a stoma. When assessing the stoma, it should appear pink/red and moist. Stool is released through the stoma, and a colostomy bag is placed to collect the stool.

GENITOURINARY DISORDERS (GU)

Assessing a Patient With Genitourinary Disorders

Review the genitourinary system in your anatomy and physiology book. Obtain a health history from the patient, assessing for any chronic or new symptoms. Assess patients for any urinary problems or prior surgeries.

Genitourinary Diagnostics

Lab Work: BUN/Cr levels and CBC.

Urinalysis and Urine Culture

KUB X-ray: X-ray images are used to view the abdomen.

Retrograde Pyelogram: Chest x-ray of the urinary tract.

Cystoscopy: A scope is used to examine the urethra and bladder.

Bladder Scan: A portable ultrasound to view the amount of urine in the bladder.

Renal Ultrasound: Images of the kidneys are viewed through ultrasound.

Urinary Tract Infection (UTIs)

Definition: This is an infection of the urinary tract, caused by bacterial organisms. Women have a shorter urethra than men, which can cause more frequent UTIs. Patients who are immobile or have an indwelling Foley catheter are also more susceptible to UTIs.

Signs and Symptoms: Burning when urinating, difficulty urinating, mental status changes in older patients, fever, abdominal cramping, incontinence, nausea, vomiting, foul-smelling urine, and urinary frequency.

Diagnostics: Urinalysis and urine culture.

Complications: Worsening of symptoms and acute pyelonephritis.

Drug Therapy: **Broad-spectrum antibiotics, sulfa drugs (assess for sulfa allergies before administering), intravenous fluids, phenazopyridine (Pyridium), and analgesics.** ←

Nursing Care: Administer medications as ordered. Monitor intake and output. Encourage PO intake. Provide Foley catheter care if patient has indwelling catheter. Perianal care is important. Instruct patient to remember to wipe from front to back. Teach patient preventative measures for patients with chronic UTIs.

Glomerulonephritis

➔ *Definition:* This is an **infection and inflammation of the glomerulus of the kidneys. It is usually caused by beta-hemolytic streptococci.**

Signs and Symptoms: Fever, edema, abdominal pain, hematuria, red-brown colored urine, shortness of breath, decreased urine output, and hypertension.

Diagnostics: Strep test, urine culture and urinalysis; BUN/Cr is increased, and protein is seen in the urine.

Complications: Chronic kidney disease.

Drug Therapy: Antibiotics, antihypertensives, analgesics, and diuretics.

Nursing Care: Fluid restriction is needed with low sodium intake. Monitor blood pressure. Assess for fluid overload and edema. Administer medications as ordered.

Nephrotic Syndrome

Definition: Nephrotic syndrome is a set of symptoms that occur because of damage to the glomerulus. It can result from glomerulonephritis.

Signs and Symptoms: Protein in the urine, blood in the urine, weight loss, edema, fever, hypertension, fatigue, and weakness.

Diagnostics: Lab work such as albumin, CBC, and CMP. CT scan of the abdomen and urine culture.

Complications: Kidney failure.

Drug Therapy: Corticosteroids, antihypertensives, diuretics, albumin, and immunosuppressant medications.

Nursing Care: Obtain a urine sample. Administer medication as ordered. Implement strict intake and output monitoring. Assess for edema. Labs should be checked daily for improvement in lab values. Continue to monitor blood pressure. Assess for signs of infection.

Pyelonephritis

Definition: This is an inflammation of the ureters and kidneys caused by bacterial infections.

Signs and Symptoms: Fever, abdominal pain, difficulty urinating, and bloody urine (hematuria).

Diagnostics: CT of abdomen and lab work.

Complications: Renal failure.

Drug Therapy: Antibiotics, antipyretics, and analgesics.

Nursing Care: Monitor vital signs. Administer medications as ordered. Monitor intake and output. Increased PO fluid intake and intravenous fluids may be needed. Monitor urine for blood. Continue to monitor for complications.

Kidney Stones

Definition: This condition is caused by buildup of calcium, oxalate, or uric acid in the kidneys, resulting in the formation of stones and changes in urine pH.

Signs and Symptoms: Difficult and painful urination, nausea, vomiting, pain in the flank area, and bloody urine.

Diagnostics: X-ray of the abdomen, KUB, pyelogram, labs, and urinalysis.

Complications: Kidney failure.

Drug Therapy: Pain medication, antiemetic, thiazide diuretics, anticholinergics, and allopurinol (Zyloprim) to decrease calcium buildup in patients with calcium-containing stones.

Nursing Care: Increase fluid intake and monitor output. Strain urine and assess to see if the patient passes the stone naturally. Monitor lab work. Administer pain medications as ordered. Surgery may be needed if patient is unable to pass the stone. Nephrolithotomy, lithotripsy, and cystoscopy with stents are surgical procedures used to remove stones. A nephrostomy tube may be inserted to protect the kidney from further damage or infection. An ileal conduit may be needed for conditions such as kidney stone, tumor, or neurogenic bladder. An ileal conduit is a urinary diversion via a stoma through which the urine is excreted into a bag.

Acute Renal Failure

Definition: Acute renal failure is rapid loss of renal function that occurs in three main stages: oliguric, diuretic, and recovery. A decrease in urine output can cause acute renal failure.

Signs and Symptoms:

- Oliguric stage: This begins with a decrease in urine output, increase in BUN/Cr, metabolic acidosis, hyponatremia, hyperkalemia, mental status changes, nausea, weight loss, fatigue, hypertension, and uremia. Labs are evaluated to confirm diagnosis.

- Diuretic stage: Increase in urine output, decrease in BUN/Cr levels, hypotension, hypovolemia, hypokalemia, and hyponatremia.
- Recovery stage: Urine output gradually returns to normal, BUN/Cr is normal, and urinary function stabilizes.

Diagnostics: BUN/Cr, estimated glomerular filtration rate (eGFR), CBC, CMP, urine culture, and electrolytes.

Drug Therapy: Each stage is treated individually. Loop diuretics are used to manage fluid overload, and kayexalate is administered to correct the potassium level in the oliguric stage. Intravenous fluids are administered in the diuretic stage. Sodium bicarbonate is administered to correct electrolyte imbalance.

Nursing Care: Ensure strict intake and output monitoring. Monitor labs and electrolytes (especially potassium), and daily weights. Administer medications as ordered. Monitor for mental status changes. Fluid restriction may be needed. Monitor for signs of UTI. The goal for patients with acute renal failure is to maintain proper kidney function. Monitor for fluid overload and assess respiratory status, urine output, and electrolytes. Patient education and emotional support are needed. Dialysis may be needed if symptoms progress or worsen.

Chronic Renal Failure

Definition: This is a progressive loss of renal function that results in end-stage renal disease if left untreated. It is caused by chronic hypertension or kidney disease. Patients with advanced disease require dialysis.

→ *Signs and Symptoms:* **Oliguria, increase in BUN/Cr, decrease in eGFR, hypervolemia, hyperkalemia, metabolic acidosis, decrease in calcium, hypertension, edema, fatigue, weight loss, changes in mental status, dry skin, tremors, pericarditis, tachypnea, nausea, stomatitis, diarrhea, hematuria, muscle weakness, and anemia.**

Diagnostics: Lab work BUN/Cr, eGFR, electrolytes, glucose levels, and renal ultrasound.

Complications: Complete loss of kidney function.

Drug Therapy: Antihypertensives, diuretics, erythropoietin (Arnesp) for anemia, phosphate binders, intravenous fluids, sodium polystyrene (Kayexalate), sodium bicarbonate, antibiotics, calcium with vitamin D, and dialysis may be needed to treat chronic kidney failure.

Nursing Care: Monitor vital signs. Closely monitor strict intake and output. Monitor for fluid overload and edema. Daily weights are monitored. Cardiac monitoring is needed. Monitor electrolytes. Elevate lower extremities. Provide skin care. Administer medications as ordered. Monitor daily labs. Provide patient education and emotional support.

Dialysis

Definition: Dialysis is a procedure that filters the body's blood by increasing the movement of fluid across a semipermeable membrane. The removal of waste products, electrolytes, and excess water through the pores of the membrane requires several hours. Dialysis is used because the kidneys no longer function and the body is unable to remove these substances on its own—think of it as a sort of car wash for the bloodstream. There are two types of dialysis, peritoneal and hemodialysis. Dialysis is typically given through an AV fistula or Quinton catheter. Labs such as BUN/Cr and GFR are monitored while the patient is on dialysis.

Types of Dialysis: Hemodialysis is the removal of waste products through a vascular access such as an arteriovenous (AV) fistula. Assess vital signs and labs before starting dialysis. Peritoneal dialysis is the removal of waste products using the patient's own peritoneal cavity, without the use of artificial membranes.

Hemodialysis Care: Hemodialysis consists of administering a dialysate through a catheter while simultaneously withdrawing blood through a separate lumen. The blood is filtered outside the body in a dialyzer machine. The vascular access can be any large vein, for example, the subclavian or femoral vein. An AV fistula offers permanent access and is most commonly used. Assess the site for any signs of infection. Patients can receive dialysis in an outpatient facility on scheduled days, such as Mondays, Wednesdays, or Fridays and/or Tuesdays, Thursdays, and Saturdays. Medications should be held until after dialysis. Blood products can be given while the patient is in dialysis. Never draw blood from the AV fistula.

Before dialysis, do a full assessment, take vital signs, monitor daily weights, assess for edema, and listen to lung sounds. The patient's weight should be taken before and after dialysis. Many patients with chronic renal failure experience anemia during dialysis, and medications such as epoetin alfa (Epogen) are used to treat it. During the infusion, assess the patient for complications and reactions. Dialysis is administered by a dialysis nurse only.

Complications of Hemodialysis:

- Muscle and abdominal cramping: If dialysate (the dialysis solution) is administered too quickly, muscle and abdominal cramping can occur. Infusing the dialysate at a slower rate can decrease the patient's discomfort.
- Hypotension: Due to the large amount of fluid removed, patients can become hypotensive during dialysis. Hanging a bag of IVF can help treat low blood pressure. Hold blood pressure medications until the dialysis procedure is complete.
- Disequilibrium syndrome: This is caused by rapid administration of dialysate. Treatment is to stop or slow the rate of the dialysate. Administer a hypertonic solution.
- Air embolus: If chest pain or chest discomfort occurs during the infusion, stop dialysis immediately. Monitor vital signs, place oxygen on the patients, and call the physician immediately. This is an emergency and needs to be treated immediately.

Peritoneal Dialysis Care: Peritoneal dialysis uses the patient's peritoneal cavity instead of an artificial membrane to drain waste products. A catheter is surgically placed in the peritoneum through which dialysate is infused and fluid withdrawn. This procedure is for long-term use, and healing of the site needs to occur before dialysis can take place. Provide site care, monitor vital signs, and assess signs for infection.

Complications of Peritoneal Dialysis:

- Infection: Strict aseptic technique is needed when dialysis is given. Infection of the site can occur, which may require removal of the catheter. Cultures of the blood or the catheter tip may be needed, as well.
- Peritonitis: Cloudy drainage from the peritoneum can signify an infection. A physician needs to be notified so antibiotics can be administered.
- Abdominal pain: This can occur during dialysis and can usually be alleviated by administering at a slow rate. Never stop the dialysis; always slow the rate first.

Kidney Transplantation

If the patient cannot tolerate hemodialysis or peritoneal dialysis, a kidney transplant may be needed. A compatible donor will be used for the transplant. Preoperative and postoperative teaching is necessary. The most important postoperative action is assessing for signs of infection or rejection of the kidney. Signs and symptoms are increased lab values, abdominal tenderness over the graft site, hypertension, fever, and a decrease in renal function. To prevent infection and rejection, an immunosuppressant such as tacrolimus (Prograf) or mycophenolate mofetil (CellCept) is given. The kidney may need to be removed if further complications occur.

MUSCULOSKELETAL DISORDERS

Assessing a Patient With Musculoskeletal Disorders

Review the musculoskeletal system in your anatomy and physiology book. Obtain a health history from the patient, assessing for any chronic or new symptoms. There are many joints, bones, and muscles in the musculoskeletal system; there is no need to memorize all of them. Become familiar with the bones and joints, as well as bones that are commonly injured. Ask patients about their mobility. Are they able to walk on their own? Do they need a walker or wheelchair? Are patients bedbound? Conduct range of motion testing; assess for any limitations, weakness, or pain. Remember that age is an important consideration when assessing a patient's musculoskeletal system.

Musculoskeletal Diagnostics

X-ray or CT scan, bone scan, labs (such as calcium level), electromyelogram (EMG), bone biopsy, MRI, and arthroscopies are some diagnostics used in musculoskeletal disorders.

Fractures

Definition: A fracture is a break or injury in a bony structure caused by an injury or fall.

Signs and Symptoms: Pain at the site, swelling, tenderness, limited mobility, muscle spasms, deformity, bruising, and bleeding at site. There are several types of fractures, including complete (completely through the bone), hairline (partially through the bone), and simple closed fractures (the bone is broken but not through the skin).

Diagnostics: X-ray, MRI, CT scan, PT/INR, and a neurovascular exam.

Complications: **Infection, DVT, compartment syndrome, fat emboli, and pulmonary embolism can occur from fractures. Compartment syndrome occurs when there is increased pressure against the muscle. Signs and symptoms are pallor, parasthesia, pain, pressure, paralysis, and pulse—the 6Ps! Fat emboli typically occur in long bone fractures such as the femur or pelvis. Fat emboli occur when fat tissue travels in the bloodstream and causes a clot. The**

symptoms of fat emboli are shortness of breath, change in mental status, respiratory failure, cyanosis, and hypoxia, and require immediate intervention. Monitor for complications.

Drug Therapy: Antibiotics, NSAIDs, muscle relaxers, narcotics, and corticosteroids.

Surgical Care: Before surgery, the patient is immobilized with traction, medications are given as ordered, intravenous fluids are administered, and the patient is prepared for surgery. Postoperative care includes, pain management, incision care, vital signs, intake and output, antibiotics, neurovascular checks, and anticoagulants. Continue to assess for complications. The most common surgery done to repair fractures is an open reduction internal fixation (ORIF), in which hardware (e.g., pins or screws) is used to mobilize the fracture. During the recovery phase, physical therapy is ordered.

Nursing Care: Administer medications as ordered; pain management, anticoagulants, and antibiotics must all be given postoperatively. Monitor vital signs. Positioning the patient is very important to provide comfort, taking note of whether the patient is weight bearing or non–weight bearing on the extremity. Neurovascular checks are done every 2 to 4 hours. Cast care is particularly important. Ensure that the cast is not wet, and teach the patient to never stick anything down the cast. Assess the skin under and around the cast for any signs of odor or infections. Drains are used to remove excess blood/fluid from the site. Types of drains are Jackson-Pratt (JP), Stryker, or Hemovac drains. Physicians are the only providers who can remove the drain. Monitor the incision site for infection, and empty drains every shift. Dressing changes are done per physician order. A Foley catheter is used to drain urine and is typically removed on postop day 1 or 2. The patient will be prescribed physical therapy. Monitor for complications.

Traction

Traction is used to immobilize a fracture, maintain alignment, and decrease muscle spasms. You will be responsible for knowing the various types of traction. Refer to your textbook for visualization of the different types of tractions. (Hint: Professors often include pictures of different types of traction on exams, so be sure you can identify them.) When traction is used, it is important to check → the neurovascular system and site for infection. **Check the extremity for numbness, color, temperature of the skin, capillary refill, edema, pulses, and pain. Continue to assess for complications that may occur.**

Types of traction:

- Buck's traction: Immobilizes the extremity while weights hang freely off the bed. Never remove weights without the physician's consent.
- Bryant's traction: Used for hip dysplasia in children younger than 3 years old.
- Skeletal traction: Pins maintain alignment of the fracture. When pin care is performed, always use aseptic techniques when cleaning the site.

Casts

There are two common types of casts—plaster and synthetic. Plaster casts take 48 hours to dry, and weight bearing is not allowed until after the cast is fully dry. Synthetic casts dry in 15 minutes, and weight bearing is allowed after 30 minutes of cast placement. Here are some important facts about casts to remember when tested:

- Petal the casts to provide a smooth edge.
- Assess the skin and neurovascular status for any complications.
- **Do not stick anything down the casts. If the skin becomes itchy, cool air can be applied to the leg to relieve symptoms.** ←
- If the patient feels warmth or pain under the cast, do a neurovascular assessment and call the physician.
- Pulmonary embolism is a major complication with fractures; continue to signs and symptoms of blood clots.

Osteoarthritis

Definition: This is a slow and progressive deterioration of bone tissue, joints, and cartilage.

Signs and Symptoms: Joint pain, joint deformity, fatigue, swelling, and limited range of motion.

Diagnostics: X-ray, CT scan, MRI, or bone scan.

Complications: Chronic pain and progressive weakness of the joint.

Drug Therapy: NSAIDs, pain relievers, COX-2 inhibitors such as Celebrex, and injected steroids.

Nursing Care: Administer medications as ordered, with pain management. Provide comfort for the patient, and provide heat to soothe joints. Instruct the patient to rest the joints periodically during the day to prevent swelling and severe pain. Physical therapy should be ordered to maintain range of motion (ROM). Assist patients with walking, and take precautions to prevent falls. If symptoms persist, a joint replacement may be needed.

Osteoporosis

Definition: Osteoporosis is a chronic and progressive bone disorder. Osteoporosis or bone loss can be caused by low calcium levels and chronic steroid use. Postmenopausal women are commonly affected.

→ *Signs and Symptoms:* Pain, loss of height, swelling in the extremity, and **frequent fractures.**

Diagnostics: Bone density test, bone scan, and serum calcium, vitamin D, and phosphorus levels.

Complications: Fractures.

Drug Therapy: Calcium supplements are given with vitamin D. Other medications such as calcitonin (Calcimar), alendronate (Fosamax), ibandronate (Boniva), and raloxifene (Evista) are used to promote healthy bone formation. NSAIDs are used to treat pain.

Nursing Care: Implement safety measures to prevent falls or fractures. Administer medications as ordered. Proper nutrition and exercise are important. People who are at risk for osteoporosis should have routine bone density tests to determine bone loss.

Osteomyelitis

Definition: Osteomyelitis is infection of the bone, tissue, or bone marrow, and is caused by *Staphylococcus aureus.*

Signs and Symptoms: Tenderness, swelling, fever, pain, nausea, chills, and sepsis.

Diagnostics: Bone aspiration and biopsy, CBC, wound culture, and blood cultures.

Complications: Sepsis.

Drug Therapy: Long-term IV antibiotics, antipyretics, and pain management.

→ *Nursing Care:* Administer IV antibiotics as ordered. **The patient may need a PICC or midline catheter inserted for the administration of long-term antibiotics.** Contact precautions need to be in place if the wound is infected. The wound may need a surgical debridement. Dressing changes are done per physician order. Continue to monitor for sepsis.

Gout

Definition: Gout is caused by calcium buildup and increased uric acid in the joints.

Signs and Symptoms: Tenderness, swelling, and pain.

Diagnostics: Lab work such as uric acid. A gout flare occurs when the uric acid is less than 6 mg/dL.

Complications: Osteoarthritis.

Drug Therapy: Antigout medications such as colchicine and allopurinol (Zyloprim).

Nursing Care: Administer medication as ordered. Putting ice to the joint may relieve pain and swelling. Encourage an increase in fluid intake. A low purine diet is recommended for patients with gout. Purine is a chemical that is found in food that breaks down into uric acid, which can lead to gout. Teach the patient avoid foods high in purine.

Rheumatoid Arthritis (RA)

Definition: This is a systemic and chronic autoimmune disease that causes inflammation of the connective tissue and synovial joints, but also has systemic effects.

Signs and Symptoms: Joint pain, swelling, stiffness, tenderness, limited joint movements, deformity of joints, fatigue, and weight loss.

Diagnostics: Synovial fluid analysis, bone scan, and increased erythrocyte sedimentation rate, which determines the presence of inflammation. C-reactive protein is used to diagnose RA.

Complications: Severe joint deformities and limited range of motion; systemic effects in patients with severe disease include eye, lung, heart, and vascular inflammation.

Drug Therapy: Disease-modifying anti-rheumatic drugs (DMARDs) such as methotrexate (Rheumatrex), etanercept (Enbrel), and adalimumab (Humira). Other medications such as NSAIDs, corticosteroids, immunosuppressants, antibiotics, and analgesics are also used.

Nursing Care: Administer medications as ordered. Teach patients to practice ROM and maintain mobility of the joints. Surgical procedures such as arthroplasty or synovectomy may be needed if symptoms worsen. Continue to assess and monitor for pain.

INTEGUMENTARY DISORDERS

Assessing a Patient With Integumentary Disorders

Review the integumentary system in your anatomy and physiology book. Obtain a health history from the patient, assessing for any chronic or new symptoms. Remember the different layers of the skin; you will be tested on this information. (Refer to Chapter 2.) The two common disorders that are tested in this section are burns and ulcers. I will discuss these two in great detail; do not disregard the other disorders.

Integumentary Diagnostics

Assess the skin for bruises, color changes, growths, infection, and lesions. Other diagnostics such as wound cultures or skin biopsies are used.

Pressure Ulcers

Definition: A pressure ulcer is an area of the skin that breaks down as a result of pressure to the skin tissue. Ulcers occur in stages, based on the layer of skin infected. Patients who are at risk for pressure ulcers are those who are immobile, incontinent, obese, malnourished, and surgical.

Signs and Symptoms: Assessment of the ulcer is based on the stage of progression of the wound.

- Stage I: The epidermis is intact, and there is mild reddening of the area.
- Stage II: The epidermis is not intact, and partial loss of skin occurs, with a blister-like wound.
- Stage III: Complete loss of the dermis and subcutaneous tissue occurs.
- Stage IV: There is severe loss of all layers of skin. Bone, muscle, and eschar may be seen.
- Unstageable: Full tissue and skin loss occurs. The skin has yellow slough and necrotic skin.

You will be responsible for knowing the different stages of pressure ulcers.

Diagnostics: Braden scale, skin assessment, and wound culture.

Complications: Infection and sepsis.

Drug Therapy: Barrier cream may be applied to the wound. A topical medication such as collagenase (Santyl) may be applied to promote wound healing.

Nursing Care: Assessing the skin, preventing bedsores, and frequent repositioning are needed to prevent ulcerations. If an ulcer is present either on admission or during the hospital stay, the wound must be measured, a photo must be taken, and the wound must be cleaned and dressed. Place the pictures and measurements in the chart. A wound care nurse may be needed to assess and treat the wound. The nurse's role is to prevent ulceration and maintain skin integrity. Interventions include frequent turning, using a sheet to lift the patient to avoid shearing, ensuring proper nutrition and adequate fluid intake, using an air mattress, keeping the skin dry, changing patients's incontinence pads every hour, and dressing wounds as ordered. A skin assessment is done every shift and documented. A wound vac may be ordered to apply to wounds if needed.

Burns

Burns are classified by the level of severity. The levels of classification will be discussed in this chapter along with nursing interventions for each. **The Rule of Nines is used to estimate the severity of burns.** ←

Classification:

- Superficial-thickness burn: The dermis is injured. The skin appears pink in color and is painful to touch. These burns heal, and little intervention is needed.
- Superficial partial-thickness burn: The entire dermis is injured. The skin appears bright red, sensitive to touch, swollen, moist, and blanched.
- Deep partial-thickness burn: Injury extends deep into the dermis. The skin appears blistered, moist, red, and sensitive. Skin grafting may be needed to decrease scarring.
- Full-thickness burn: All layers of the skin are injured. The skin appears hard and leathery, with a waxy appearance, and may be black or yellow in color. Eschar may be noted. The skin is painless due to sensory damage. Skin grafting is necessary, and scarring may still be present afterward. Healing may take weeks or months.

Phases of Burn Injury

Emergent Phase

The emergent phase occurs within 24 to 72 hours of the burn. Preventing hypovolemic shock is important during this phase. ← Maintain a patent airway, and monitor vital signs closely. A full assessment is done, including the injured area. Hematocrit levels are decreased during this phase. Fluid resuscitation is very important, and intravenous fluids are given immediately. The consensus formula is used to determine the amount of fluids needed for the body surface burned. Become familiar with the consensus formula; you will be tested on this. A Foley catheter is inserted to monitor strict output. An NGT may also be placed to prevent aspiration, and the patient will remain NPO.

Acute Phase

In the acute phase pain management, nutrition, wound care, and prevention of infection are important. Administer pain medications as ordered. Narcotics such as hydromorphone (Diauldid) or morphine are commonly used to control pain. A benzodiazepine such as lorazepam (Ativan) is used to decrease anxiety. Assess pain using a numeric scale. Assess vital signs.

Wound care consists of skin grafting to reduce scarring and increase healing time. Autograft is the most common type of grafting and uses the patient's own skin to repair the damaged areas. Autograft is a surgical procedure in which general anesthesia is used. Postoperatively, the site is immobilized for 5 to 7 days with strict bed rest. Proper nutrition, hydration, and medications are maintained to facilitate proper healing. If the patient is unable to use his or her own skin, a donor may be needed.

Rehabilation Phase

Rehab is the last in the phases of burns. Although a difficult stage, the patient begins to have a positive hope that recovery is near. In this stage, the nurse usually works with a physical therapist to help regain strength and independence. The second important part of the rehab phase is patient education and wound care. Teach the patient to assess the wound for infection, maintain proper nutrition and fluid intake, and give medications as ordered.

Psoriasis

Definition: Chronic inflammation of the skin.

Signs and Symptoms: Skin appears red, flaky, and scaly.

Diagnostics: Based on the presentation of symptoms.

Complications: Worsening of symptoms.

Drug Therapy: Topical corticosteroids and medications such as Humira or Remicade are used. Stelara is new medication used to treat psoriasis.

Nursing Care: Apply topical corticosteroids and keep skin moist. Administer an antihistamine for the itchiness.

Methicillin-Resistant *Staphylococcus aureus* (MRSA)

Definition: This is a staph infection of the skin or wound. It is highly contagious, and contact precautions are needed when treating patients with MRSA.

Signs and Symptoms: Fever, infection, and irritation of the skin.

Diagnostics: Wound culture or nasal swab.

Complications: Sepsis and worsening of infection.

Drug Therapy: Long-term antibiotics such as IV vancomycin.

Nursing Care: MRSA is contagious, and contact precautions need to be maintained. Administer antibiotics as ordered. Pregnant women should not care for patients with MRSA. The older population is susceptible to MRSA, and patients who are transferred from nursing homes or assisted living facilities are swabbed during admission.

Cellulitis

Definition: Cellulitis is inflammation of the skin often caused by *Staphylococcus streptococcus,* or *Haemophilus influenzae.*

Signs and Symptoms: Redness at the site, pain, swelling, and fever.

Diagnostics: Wound culture and presentation of symptoms.

Complications: Worsening of symptoms.

Drug Therapy: IV antibiotics and pain medications.

Nursing Care: Administer medications as ordered. Elevate infected extremity. Use a numeric scale to assess pain.

IMMUNOLOGICAL DISORDERS

Assessing a Patient With Immunological Disorders

Review the immunological system in your anatomy and physiology book. Obtain a health history from the patient, assessing for any chronic or new symptoms. Review the immune response, immunoglobulins, and hypersensitivity reactions in your textbook. I will not discuss all the disorders in this chapter, only the most commonly tested: lupus and HIV/AIDS. Do not disregard the other information from this section; refer to your textbook or class notes for details on other disorders.

Lupus

Definition: Lupus is a genetic or systemic autoimmune disorder that attacks the major organs in the body. The cause is unknown.

Signs and Symptoms: The most common symptom is fatigue. Other symptoms are a butterfly rash, cardiac arrhythmias, seizures, anemia, mouth sores, pleural effusions, weight changes, and fever.

Diagnostics: CBC, urine analysis, chest x-ray, EKG, positive anti-DNA Smith antigen and antinuclear antibodies, and lupus erythematosus cell preparation.

Complications: Pericarditis, thrombocytopenia, lupus nephritis, and leukopenia.

Drug Therapy: Immunosuppressant medications such as cyclophosphamide (Cytoxan), NSAIDs, and corticosteroids.

Nursing Care: Administer medications as ordered. Monitor weight, vital signs, and signs of inflammation. Encourage rest to conserve energy. Maintain good nutrition and fluid intake. Assess pain and medicate as ordered.

HIV/AIDS

Definition: With this disease, there is damage to the immune system that decreases the body's CD4 T cells. It is caused by the ribonucleic acid virus, which destroys the CD4 T cells. The severity of HIV/AIDS is determined by the damage to the CD4 T-cell count. Transmission of the virus can be through sexual activity, needles, blood products, fluid exchange, and from HIV-infected mothers.

Signs and Symptoms: The patient may be asymptomatic for 10 years with no distinguishing symptoms present. Symptoms are diarrhea, weight loss, fever, shingles, cough, and fatigue. Due to the immunocompromised state, these patients are susceptible to viruses and are frequently sick. Early detection of HIV/AIDS can decrease the severity of the virus.

➔ *Diagnostics:* **Rapid HIV test, enzyme immunoassay, and western blot test. Labs such as CD4 count, CBC, and CMP are usually ordered, and urine samples may be obtained for analysis.**

Complications: Pneumonia and death if left untreated.

Drug Therapy: Antiretroviral therapy is used to treat AIDS/HIV. Treatment includes nucleotide reverse transcriptase inhibitors such as zidovudine (ZDV), abacavir (Ziagen), emtricitabine (Emtriva), and didanosine (Videx). Nonnucleoside reverse transcriptase inhibitors include nevirapine (Viramune), efavirenz (Sustiva), and delavirdine (Rescriptor). Protease inhibitors and fusion inhibitors are also used. In view of the increased risk of infection, patients should receive flu and pneumonia vaccines every year.

Nursing Care: Early detection is best; patients who are sexually active should be tested. Once diagnosed, it is important to start antiretroviral therapy immediately. Teach patients the side effects that occur with these medications. Counseling may be needed to enhance coping mechanisms. Prevention of infection is important. Malnutrition is common in these patients; maintain a high-calorie diet if needed. Education about safe sex and methods to decrease transmission is key to preventing transmission of the virus.

ONCOLOGICAL DISORDERS

Assessing a Patient With Oncological Disorders

Obtain a health history from the patient, assessing for any chronic or new symptoms. Prevention of cancer is important. Risk factors for cancer include smoking, processed foods, sun exposure, stress, and alcohol intake, and guidelines have been published outlining timing of recommended checkups. Women should receive a Pap test or breast exam and men should receive a rectal exam, colonoscopy, and testicular exam at recommended intervals. I will discuss the major types of cancer in this chapter along with treatments and interventions. The most frequently tested information involves the prevention of cancer and treatment methods. Some forms of cancer are hereditary, and identifying genetic risk factors has become a focus of research.

Oncological Diagnostics

PET scan, CT scan, MRI, biopsy, and lab work.

Detection of Cancer: Self-examinations, regular early check-ups, and early detection are all important in treating cancer. Each patient may present with different symptoms, but there are some hallmark symptoms that may help with the early detection of cancer. These are just common signs of cancer. Signs are moles that change in size, a consistent cough, significant weight loss, loss of appetite, weakness, unusual bleeding, difficulty swallowing, palpating a mass or lump, change in bowel pattern, and fever. If at any time these signs occur and become worse over time, it is time for a checkup.

Lung Cancer

Pathophysiology: Smoking is the main cause of lung cancer. There are two main types of lung cancer: small cell and non-small cell.

In both, tumors are present in the lung and often the cancer has spread elsewhere (e.g., the brain) by the time of diagnosis.

Diagnostics: Chest x-ray, CT of the chest, MRI, CBC, and bronchoscopy are used to diagnose lung cancer. In bronchoscopy, a biopsy of the tissue is taken and tested for malignancy.

Signs and Symptoms: Respiratory distress, cough, diminished breath sounds, chest pain, fever, chills, weight loss, and blood-tinged sputum.

Drug Therapy: Bronchodilators, analgesics, and corticosteroids. Radiation and chemotherapy will be administered as well. Surgical removal of the tumor may be performed.

Surgical Care: Thoracotomy, lobectomy, and thoracentesis may be performed to remove the tumor and fluid from the lung. Preoperative teaching is necessary. Postoperatively, chest tube care, IV administration, pain management, vital signs, infection prevention, and assessing for respiratory status are done. Assess the incisional site, perform dressing changes, and monitor drainage every shift.

Nursing Care: Monitor the patient's respiratory status. Administer O_2 and place the patient in high Fowler's position. Maintain a high-protein/high-calorie diet. Monitor shortness of breath and limit activity. Provide frequent rest periods. Monitor for infections. The patient may need emotional support during this time.

Breast Cancer

→ *Pathophysiology:* Here, **cancerous cells occur on the mammary ducts and are invasive or in situ.** Cancer cells can also invade the lymph nodes.

Signs and Symptoms: Palpable mass on breast, pain, nipple discharge, nipple retraction, skin retraction, and changes in breast color.

Diagnostics: Breast biopsy and sentinel lymph node dissection. Mammogram and ultrasound of the breast are used for screening and diagnosis.

Drug Therapy: Chemotherapy, such as cyclophosphamide (Cytoxan) and methotrexate (Trexall), is used to destroy cancer cells. Radiation is used to shrink the tumor. Hormonal medications such as estrogen and tamoxifen are administered. Antiemetics are used to treat nausea. Pain medication may be used.

Surgical Care: A mastectomy or lumpectomy may be performed to remove cancer cells. Never use the upper extremity for blood pressure, IVs, or lab draws from patients who have received mastectomies. A "restricted extremity" armband needs to be placed on the affected site.

Nursing Care: Yearly mammograms are recommended to prevent breast cancer. Self-exams should be performed monthly. Side effects of the medications should be discussed with the patient. Administer medications as ordered. Encourage good nutrition. Monitor for weight loss.

Colon Cancer

Pathophysiology: Adenocarcinoma is the most common type of colorectal cancer. Tumors are present on the colon.

Signs and Symptoms: Change in stool (bloody), abdominal pain, weight loss, weakness, nausea, and vomiting.

Diagnostics: Colonoscopy, CT of the abdomen, occult stool, CBC, and biopsy of colorectal polyps.

Drug Therapy: Surgery is often first-line treatment. Chemotherapy is also used to treat colon cancer, and leucovorin and fluorouracil (5-FU) are commonly used.

Surgical Care: A colon resection is performed to remove the tumor from the colon. A colostomy or ileostomy may be surgically placed as a diversion. Pain management, antibiotics, antiemetics, and antipyretics are given postoperatively.

Nursing Care: Preoperative teaching includes bowel preparation before surgery. Administer antibiotics before and after surgery. A colostomy bag is placed over the stoma, and output must be recorded every shift. Colostomy teaching is needed. Emotional support is needed. Prepare the patient for chemotherapy or radiation if needed.

Prostate Cancer

Pathophysiology: Prostate cancer commonly occurs in men aged 50 and older. It is a slow-growing cancer that can spread through the lymphatic system and bloodstream. Smoking and high-fat diet are risk factors.

Signs and Symptoms: Usually asymptomatic but patients may have bloody urine, difficulty urinating, or back pain.

Diagnostics: Labs such as prostate-specific antigen (PSA), rectal exam, biopsy of the prostate gland.

Drug Therapy: Hormonal medications are prescribed to slow tumor progression. Luteinizing hormone-releasing hormones such as leuprolide (Lupron) and goserelin (Zoladex) are often used. Pain management and corticosteroids are also administered. Chemotherapy may be administered as well. Surgical removal of the tumor may be performed.

Surgical Care: Prostatectomy may be performed to remove the tumor. A suprapubic prostatectomy or transurethral prostatectomy may be performed. After surgery, a catheter is placed, and a balloon is inflated to 30 mL to maintain hemostasis. A three-way irrigation Foley is inserted to prevent clots and allow flushing of the bladder.

Nursing Care: Monitor vital signs. If the patient has a three-way Foley in place, assess urine output and any signs of clots. If abdominal pain or a decrease in urine output occurs, call the physician. Continuous bladder irrigation decreases clotting and helps restore bladder function. Daily dressing changes are performed. Administer medications as ordered. Assess for complications.

Multiple Myeloma

Pathophysiology: Abnormal plasma cells target bone marrow, lymph nodes, spleen, liver, lungs, adrenal glands, kidneys, and skin.

Signs and Symptoms: Headache, vision changes, bone pain, weakness, change in urinary function, confusion, anemia, increased calcium and protein levels.

Diagnostics: Bone marrow aspiration, x-ray, urinalysis, and bone scan. Labs show elevation in ESR, Ca, protein, and uric acid levels.

Drug Therapy: Bone marrow transplantation and chemotherapy are used to treat multiple myeloma. Blood transfusions and platelet transfusion may be needed as well. Administer pain medication and analgesics.

Nursing Care: Monitor signs of infection, bleeding, and fractures. The patient should increase fluid intake. Education on side effects of chemotherapy should be given to the patient. Education on bone marrow biopsy and transplantation should also be provided. Monitor vital signs and assess for pain. Emotional support is needed for both patient and family.

Chemotherapy

Definition: There are various types of chemotherapy that are used to kill cancerous cells, often as they are in the process of replicating. Chemotherapy decreases the number of cancerous cells in the body, but does not always eliminate them completely. It is highly toxic and kills both abnormal (i.e., cancerous) cells and normal cells that undergo frequent cell division, such as those of the GI tract, as the drug cannot differentiate between the two. Chemotherapy has many side effects and is administered through an IV or Port-a-Cath. A Port-a-Cath allows for vascular access through the subclavian port. Use aseptic technique when accessing the port. The various types of chemotherapy are discussed in Chapter 5.

Side Effects: Many side effects occur with chemotherapy. Remember cancerous cells and normal cells are both targeted. The common side effects are weakness, fatigue, nausea, vomiting, alopecia, weight loss, diarrhea, stomatitis, impotence, anemia, thrombocytopenia, and neutropenia.

Complications: Tumor lysis syndrome is triggered by chemotherapy. Rapid destruction of tumor cells can cause severe electrolyte changes. The four main symptoms of tumor lysis syndrome are hyperkalemia, hyperphosphatemia, hyperuricemia, and hypocalcemia. Continue to assess for complications.

Nursing Care: It is important to prepare and teach the patient about chemotherapy. Discuss side effects, type, and complications. Monitor weight loss and encourage proper nutrition. Supplements may need to be given. Treat nausea and vomiting. Administer pain medications as needed. Due to the decrease in WBCs, patients are advised to wear masks when in public areas, avoid large groups, and limit visitors to reduce their risk of infection. Place signs on the patient's door that instruct staff and visitors to use precautions when entering the room. Chemotherapy precautions are also in place. Special disposal of urine and bodily fluids should be performed. Chemotherapy gloves need to be worn.

Radiation

Definition: Radiation destroys cancerous cells, and works at targeting one area of the disease. There is less damage to normal cells than with chemotherapy.

Side Effects: Radiation burns, loss of hair, change in skin pigmentation, nausea, vomiting, weight loss, radiation pneumonitis, and pericarditis.

Types of Administration:

- External beam (teletherapy): Administered over a period of 4 to 6 weeks. It is often given daily, with the total radiation dosage divided over many doses. External beam is given outside the skin and directed to the site of the tumor.
- Internal beam (brachytherapy): Radiation beam is inserted and applied directly to the tumor site. With this type of therapy, the patient releases radioactive materials, and precautions should be used. Pregnant women and children should not visit patients receiving this type of therapy. Visitors should stay for only 30 minutes or less.

Nursing Care: Protective wear is necessary when taking care of patients receiving internal beam radiation. Wear gloves, dispose of urine and bodily fluids using protective wear, and never use bare hands to care for a patient. Assess for side effects and treat as ordered.

HEMATOLOGICAL DISORDERS

Sickle Cell Anemia

Definition: This is a condition involving abnormal hemoglobin that results in sickled red blood cells, which can obstruct blood vessels and are more likely to targeted for cell destruction. It is an inherited autosomal recessive disorder.

Signs and Symptoms: Pain, dehydration, decrease in hemoglobin and hematocrit, fever, visual disturbances, weakness, and fatigue.

Diagnostics: Labs such as hemoglobin, hematocrit, erythrocyte, and sickle turbidity test.

Complications: Sequestration crisis.

Drug Therapy: Pain management, oxygen, IV fluids, and blood transfusion.

Nursing Care: Controlling pain and administering oxygen, intravenous fluids, and blood transfusion help treat a sickle cell crisis. Heat can be applied to the area of pain. Maintain rest periods. Patients are at risk for narcotic abuse, and teaching should be done to promote other methods to control pain when symptoms flare.

Hemophilia

Definition: Hemophilia is a clotting disorder. There are two types: hemophilia A (factor VIII deficiency) and hemophilia B (factor IX deficiency).

Signs and Symptoms: Bruising, nosebleeds, swollen/edematous joints, and blood in stool or urine.

Diagnostics: Factor assay and lab work (PTT, PT, and INR)

Complications: Intracranial hemorrhage or GI bleed.

Drug Therapy: Desmopressin (DDAVP) and factor VIII of IX concentrate.

Nursing Care: These patients are at high risk of bleeding. Teach the patient to use caution when brushing teeth or shaving. Monitor for signs of bleeding.

Myelodysplastic Syndrome (MDS)

Definition: This disease is associated with a decrease in the production of bone marrow and red blood cells.

Signs and Symptoms: Anemia, weakness, shortness of breath, and risk of bleeding.

Diagnostics: Lab work and bone marrow examination.

Complications: Bleeding and severe decrease in hemoglobin and hematocrit.

Drug Therapy: Blood and platelet transfusion, oxygen, and intravenous fluids.

Nursing Care: Patients with MDS are transfused weekly or monthly on an outpatient basis. When blood cell counts are extremely low, hospitalization is needed. Cross-match and transfusion precautions are taken.

These patients are fatigued and weak; use fall precautions.

Disseminated Intravascular Coagulation (DIC)

Definition: This is a clotting disorder in which numerous clots can form in small vessels throughout the body.

Signs and Symptoms: Ecchymosis, easy bruising, hypotension, and thrombocytopenia.

Diagnostics: Lab work (PT, PTT, INR).

Complications: Shock and sepsis.

Drug Therapy: Platelet transfusion and anticoagulant therapy.

Nursing Care: These patients are at risk for clots. Assess for complications. Administer anticoagulants as ordered. Administer oxygen if needed. Administer platelets.

Finally! We have completed the medical–surgical chapter. I know this chapter has tons of information and things to remember, which probably feels overwhelming right now. Keep in mind that these are the most common disorders, diseases, and conditions you will see in your nursing career. This course is very important, and the information taught in this class will be used not only in school but in your nursing career as well. Take each section, and work through it as best you can. Write the information down on notecards, create a sheet for each disorder or category, or use whatever method works for you. You will pass this course, and yes, it will take lots of studying. Attend study groups—they help!

Remember this study guide is designed to be used along with your class notes and textbook. I have highlighted the most commonly tested disorders in this chapter. Follow your syllabus, and study the other disorders that are highlighted in class. Keep your notes for this course; typically, this course is divided into two parts, and the final course of nursing school combines all the information. Use the notes from this class to help you study and pass the final exam. It will be helpful on the NCLEX, as well. Now, take a break before moving on to pharmacology—you deserve it.

FOUR

EMERGENCY NURSING

Emergency nursing is needed when a patient presents with a critical illness or medical situation. As nurses, our job is to prevent complications, but not all critical situations can be prevented. It is part of our job to quickly respond to these situations and treat immediately. You may have a situation where a rapid response or code blue is called, meaning that a patient's current medical status has changed from stable to critical. A critical care team is available to provide care in these situations, where a quick response is key to patients' survival. In this chapter, I discuss the most common emergency situations you may encounter as a nursing student and as a nurse. When you begin your preceptorship or new grad program, make sure you know where to locate the crash cart, how to perform CPR, and how to recognize when a patient is on the decline. Nurses are often the ones to recognize when a patient is in need of immediate care.

Cardiac Arrest

Definition: The sudden blockage of blood flow to the heart and oxygen to the brain.

Signs and Symptoms: The symptoms that can occur beforehand are dizziness, loss of consciousness, chest pain, arrhythmias, and shortness of breath.

Drug Therapy: Epinephrine, atropine, and amiodarone are used.

Nursing Interventions: Call a code! Initiate CPR immediately. Once the patient is resuscitated, he or she is transferred to the ICU for further treatment and care. The patient may be intubated as well. Administer medication as ordered by the emergency care physician. An implantable cardioverter defibrillator is used to prevent cardiac arrest.

Septic Shock

Definition: A life-threatening complication in which infections travel through the bloodstream, infecting multiple organs in the body. It is a systemic infection with multisystem effects that can cause a patient to crash rapidly.

Signs and Symptoms: Severe fever, increase in heart rate, decrease in blood pressure, change in mental status, shortness of breath, and abdominal pain.

Diagnostics: Blood cultures may be obtained.

Nursing Interventions: To treat a decrease in blood pressure, a bolus of intravenous saline will be given rapidly. Continue to monitor blood pressure closely. Vasopressors will be administered to help increase the blood pressure. Intravenous antibiotics are administered. If septic shock occurs, call the physician immediately.

Hypertensive Crisis

Definition: A severe increase in blood pressure that can range from 200/120 to 180/120. An increased blood pressure can lead to stroke and can cause organ damage.

Signs and Symptoms: Nausea, vomiting, severe anxiety, shortness of breath, seizures, chest pain, severe headache, blurred vision, and loss of consciousness.

Nursing Interventions: IV medications to decrease blood pressure are given. A continuous drip may be needed to decrease blood pressure. Once the blood pressure is reduced, treat the other underlying issues. Diuretics are used to decrease fluid overload.

Perforated Bowel

Definition: An opening that occurs in the large or small intestine, which can lead to peritonitis. This is a medical emergency, and surgery is needed immediately.

Signs and Symptoms: Severe abdominal pain, chills, change in mental status, nausea, vomiting, fever, increased heart rate, and shortness of breath.

Nursing Interventions: Surgery, temporary colostomy, and aggressive antibiotics are needed. A patient may be placed in an induced coma until symptoms are resolved and the patient is stabilized.

Gastrointestinal Bleed

Definition: A GI bleed can occur in the upper or lower tract. Causes are ulcers, cancers, or hemorrhoids. This is not always considered a medical emergency, but can quickly become an emergency due to rapid loss of blood.

Signs and Symptoms: Occult blood in the stool, weakness, dizziness, fainting, hypotension, rapid fluid loss, increased heart rate, and loss of consciousness.

Diagnostics: Occult stool sample and monitoring of hemoglobin/hematocrit levels. A colonoscopy may be needed to determine the cause of bleeding.

Drug Therapy: Vasopressors are used to treat hypotension.

Nursing Interventions: A loss of consciousness may occur due to the rapid loss of blood. These patients are on strict bed rest. A bedpan must be used until the blood levels have stabilized. Administer intravenous fluids and blood transfusions.

Ileus

Definition: Paralysis of the GI tract caused by a bowel obstruction.

Signs and Symptoms: Abdominal distension, abdominal pain, vomiting, and severe constipation.

Diagnostics: CT scan of the abdomen.

Drug Therapy: Antibiotics and intravenous fluids.

Nursing Care: An untreated ileus can cause a complete loss of GI function. A nasogastric tube is needed to decompress the intestines and treat severe vomiting. Administer parenteral nutrition. Administer pain medications as needed.

Diabetic Ketoacidosis

Definition: This occurs when there is a increase in blood glucose to a critical level and ketones enter the bloodstream.

Signs and Symptoms: Confusion, shortness of breath, excessive thirst, abdominal pain, fatigue, and weakness.

Diagnostics: Urine sample and blood glucose levels.

Nursing Interventions: Obtain blood glucose and ketones levels. Administer intravenous fluids as ordered. Patients may require an insulin drip to decrease blood glucose levels. Monitor blood glucose levels closely and frequently. Diabetic teaching is needed.

Respiratory Failure

Definition: A lack of gas exchange that causes an increase in carbon dioxide levels.

Signs and Symptoms: Loss of consciousness, shortness of breath, hypoxemia, increased respirations, and critical changes in arterial blood gases.

Diagnostics: Arterial blood gases.

Nursing Interventions: CPR is initiated. Mechanical ventilation is needed. A respiratory stimulant such as doxapram is given. As symptoms start to resolve, mechanical ventilation is slowly withdrawn.

FIVE

PHARMACOLOGY

Oh, pharmacology! One of the many responsibilities of a nurse is to safely administer medication to patients. It is important to know what you are administering, its side effects, and the route. You should also be able to educate the patient on the medications prescribed. With that said, as you look at the syllabus for this course, you may be asking yourself, "How am I supposed to learn all these medications?" or "Should I run for the door now?" Don't run, and there is no hiding! I am not going to lie or sugarcoat anything: This course was very difficult for me. I used my textbook, class notes, and other study guides to help me get through the course, but even with these resources it was a little bit of a struggle. I was able to come up with different methods to help me with each medication, which I will explain later in this chapter.

Now in retrospect, I have figured out a way to share with you that can make this course a little easier. Take each section and study it individually instead of cramming all the information together. This is not a course that you can study for the night before the exam. This is information you will need now and throughout your career. Take each system, and learn the medications for each group individually. One week, study the cardiovascular system medications, and the next week, study the medications used in the gastrointestinal system. Every day, review and learn a medication, including its side effects and nursing interventions. By the end of the week, you should know the medications for each system. Also, I have provided little tips to help you remember the medications.

Medications have a trade and a generic name. It is important to become familiar with both. Yes, it is important to memorize, but by learning to recognize the endings of many medications, you will be able to identify what class they belong to, and thus what they are used to treat. Consider the drug atenolol/Tenormin (the trade name is always capitalized). The ending "–olol" is used in the generic names of almost all beta-blockers used to treat hypertension and tachycardia. So, other medications such as metoprolol/Lopressor or carvedilol/Coreg would treat what disorder? You got it! Hypertension/tachycardia. Pay attention to the hints I have provided for you. Use this study guide along with the class notes and textbook. There are also many phone apps that can help you with medications as well. Nurses are always using medication guides to look up medications and education sheets for patients. So get those medication guides out and let's get started!

A LITTLE PHARMACOLOGY ADVICE

There is some underlying information that needs to be addressed before we jump into chatting about administering medications. The format of this chapter is structured to define each medication, list its side effects, explain its pharmacokinetics, and summarize related nursing care. Administering medication is no joke, and should be taken very seriously. Giving the wrong medication can cause severe reactions or harm to patients. So it is very important to learn and apply the five rights of patient safety and know what you are giving and why. Carry a drug guidebook or app on your phone to help look up medications. The world of medication is huge, and new medications are being introduced all the time. Do not feel embarrassed to look up meds; as nurses, we all do it. It is almost impossible to remember what all the medications are used for.

In the hospital, medications are administered electronically. The patient wears an armband that is scanned and registered into the computer. This is a great process because there is less room for error. Before administering medications, you should know what the medication treats. Always look at parameters when administering. Blood pressure medications should be given after a blood pressure reading has been taken. Typically, when the blood pressure is less than 100, the blood pressure medication is held. Assess the patient's ability to swallow before administering a medication. *Always* assess for drug allergies before administering any medication. Does the patient have a percutaneous endoscopic gastrostomy (PEG) tube through which medications are given? This will all be discussed in clinical. The exams were designed to test each medication based on the different review of systems. Frequently tested are the names of medications, what they are used to treat, and side effects. Review your syllabus and class notes for more exam info.

SAFE MEDICATION ADMINISTRATION

The Five Rights of Patient Safety

1. The right patient
2. The right drug/medication

3. The right dose
4. The right route
5. The right time

The Six Rights of Medication Administration

1. Right written or electronic order
2. Right route and dose
3. Right to have access to information
4. Right to have policies of medication
5. Right to administer medications safely
6. Right to stop and think about medications

Ways to Prevent Medication Errors

1. Have knowledge about the medication (e.g., does it interact with foods, or does the medication fall within parameters).
2. Before administration, scan the patient, and match the medication to the patient.
3. State what medication you are administering and the dose to the patient.
4. Be aware of the side effects and adverse reactions to medications.

PHARMACOKINETICS

Definition: Movement of medication through the body, including how the drug is metabolized and excreted in the body. In simple terms, pharmacokinetics is how the drug works in the body, and this is divided into four processes—absorption, distribution, metabolism, and excretion.

- Absorption: The rate at which the drug travels into the bloodstream, and how the medication is given. There are four main routes: intravenous, intramuscular, subcutaneous, and oral. Administering medications via IV is the fastest route of administration.
- Distribution: This relates to how the medication flows through the body by way of the vascular system and tissues. In order for a medication to take effect, it must be distributed and metabolized.
- Metabolism: This is the process by which the body breaks down the medication in preparation for excretion. Most medications are metabolized by the liver or kidney. Metabolism takes place by means of the enzyme CYP450 system. Many factors can affect the rate at which a medication is metabolized.
- Excretion: This is the process by which the body eliminates the medication, typically through the urine. Medications

are excreted from the body through several organs (e.g., the lungs, GI tract, various glands) but especially by the kidneys, via glomerular filtration.

PHARMACODYNAMICS

Definition: Basically, what the drugs do in the body and how they do it.

Drug–Receptor Relationship: Think of this as a real relationship. The drug binds to the receptor that leads to a response. There are several types of receptors that promote responses. Some are positive, and others are negative.

Therapeutic Dosage: Therapeutic dosage refers to the amount of the drug needed to produce the desired or therapeutic results. The therapeutic index is often used to determine the therapeutic dosage. **Remember that a medication with a low therapeutic index is not safe.**

CARDIOVASCULAR MEDICATIONS

Antihypertensive Drugs

Definition: **Antihypertensive medications decrease blood pressure and pulse by excreting sodium/water and decreasing cardiac output.** These medications treat hypertension, tachycardia, and edema.

Types: Beta-blockers, calcium channel blockers (CCBs), angiotensin-converting enzyme inhibitors (ACE inhibitors), diuretics, and angiotensin II receptor blockers (ARBs).

I. Diuretics: Thiazides, Loop, and Potassium Sparing

Thiazides

Definition: Thiazides decrease blood pressure and edema by excreting sodium and water.

Types: Hydrochlorothiazide (Hydrodiuril), chlorothiazide (Diuril), and metolazone (Zaroxolyn) are commonly used.

Contraindication: Patients with hypotension or renal failure.

Pharmacokinetics: Metabolized and excreted through the kidneys.

Side Effects: Hypokalemia, hyponatremia, hypotension, dehydration, hyperglycemia, hyperuricemia, and orthostatic hypotension.

Nursing Care: Obtain blood pressure and pulse before administering. Continue to monitor potassium levels. Monitor output. Administered by mouth (PO).

Loop Diuretics

Definition: These are the most effective of the diuretics. Loop diuretics reduce sodium and water in the loop of Henle to decrease edema, fluid overload, and hypertension. Typically given to patients who have CHF, edema, or hypertension.

Types of Loop Diuretics: Furose**mide** (Lasix), torse**mide** (Demadex), and bumetanide (Bumex).

Contraindication: Patients who have hypokalemia, hypotension, or renal failure.

Pharmacokinetics: Metabolized and excreted by the kidneys.

Side Effects: Dehydration, hearing loss, hypokalemia, hyponatremia, hypocalcemia, increase in uric acid, and hypotension.

Nursing Care: Obtain vital signs before administering. Monitor BP before and after. Monitor electrolytes. Obtain daily weights. Monitor urine output. **If patient is experiencing shortness of breath or if crackles in lung are heard on auscultation, Lasix is usually administered IV push.** Assess for output to see if the medication is effective. Can be given IV or orally. **Pay attention to the "–mide" ending (which indicates a loop diuretic).** ←

Potassium-Sparing Diuretics

Definition: These are diuretics in which potassium is spared and excretion of sodium and water is increased to reduce edema and fluid overload.

Types: Spironolactone (Aldactone), eplerenone (Inspra), and triamterene (Dyrenium).

Contraindications: Patients who suffer from kidney failure.

Pharmacokinetics: Metabolized and excreted through the kidneys.

Side Effects: Hyperkalemia, nausea, dehydration, and dizziness.

Nursing Care: Monitor potassium levels and output.

II. Beta-Adrenergic Blockers (Beta-Blockers): All -olol, -ilol, -alol Endings

Definition: Beta-blockers decrease cardiac output by releasing norepinephrine, epinephrine, and catecholamine to decrease blood pressure. They are used for patients with hypertension, myocardial infarction, and dysthymias.

Types: Aten**olol** (Tenormin), nebiv**olol** (Bystolic), metopr**olol** (Lopressor), propan**olol** (Inderal), labet**olol** (Trandate), carved**ilol** (Coreg), nald**olol** (Corgard), acebut**olol** (Sectral), and bisopr**olol** (Zebeta).

Contraindications: Patients with low blood pressure, heart failure, bradycardia, bronchospasms, and renal disease. → **Patients with diabetes mellitus should use beta-blockers with caution because these medications may mask signs of hypoglycemia.**

Pharmacokinetics: Metabolized by the liver and excreted in the urine.

Side Effects: Bradycardia, hypotension, dizziness, dry mouth, hyperglycemia, fatigue, nausea, bronchospasms, nightmares, and insomnia.

Nursing Care: Before administering these medications, assess vital signs. Follow parameters before administering dosage. Monitor side effects. Assess for orthostatic hypotension or signs of → decreased blood pressure. **Patients who take beta-blockers should use caution when taking over-the-counter medications.**

III. Calcium Channel Blockers (CCBs): All -dipine Endings

Definition: These medications decrease cardiac contractility by inhibiting calcium ions. CCBs are used to promote dilation of the blood vessels, which results in a decrease in blood pressure. They are used for patients with hypertension, dysrhythmias, and angina.

Types: amlo**dipine** (Norvasc), nife**dipine** (Procardia), diltiazem (Cardizem), verapamil (Calan), and clevi**dipine** (Cleviprex).

Contraindications: Patients with hypotension, congestive heart failure, and atrioventricular block.

Pharmacokinetics: Metabolized and excreted by the liver.

Side Effects: Dizziness, constipation, hypotension, edema, headaches, bradycardia, and gingival hyperplasia.

Nursing Care: Obtain a set of vital signs before administering medication. Follow parameters if ordered by the physician. Monitor for side effects.

IV. Angiotensin-Converting Enzyme Inhibitors: All "-pril" Endings

Definition: ACE inhibitors are used to prevent the conversion of angiotensin I to angiotensin II to increase cardiac output and contractility.

Types: lisino**pril** (Zestril), capto**pril** (Capoten), benza**pril** (Lotensin), enala**pril** (Vasotec), rami**pril** (Altace), and quina**pril** (Accupril).

Contraindications: Patients with hypotension, MI, renal and heart failure.

Pharmacokinetics: Metabolized and excreted by the kidneys.

Side Effects: **Persistent dry cough, orthostatic hypotension, loss of taste, hyperkalemia, renal failure, dizziness, and tachycardia.** ←

Nursing Care: Obtain a set of vital signs before administering medication. Follow parameters if ordered by the physician. Monitor for side effects such as persistent cough; consider changing medication if symptoms persist. Monitor patients' renal function while they are on these medications.

V. Angiotensin II Receptor Blockers: All "-sartan" Endings

Definition: These medications block angiotensin II receptors, resulting in a decrease in blood pressure. Used to treat hypertension.

Types: lor**sartan** (Cozaar), val**sartan** (Diovan), olme**sartan** (Benicar), irbe**sartan** (Avapro), telmi**sartan** (Micardis), cande**sartan** (atacand), azil**sartan** (Edarbi), and epro**sartan** (Teveten).

Contraindications: Patients who are hypotensive.

Pharmacokinetics: Metabolized and excreted by the kidneys.

Side Effects: Hypotension, dizziness, tachycardia, nausea, and hypoglycemia.

Nursing Care: Obtain vital signs before administering dose. ARBs and ACE inhibitors are given together for patients who suffer from severe dry cough. Monitor blood glucose levels. Report any side effects to the physician.

Cholesterol-Lowering Medications/ Antihyperlipidemic Medications

I. HMG-CoA Reductase Inhibitors: All "–statin" Endings

Definition: Known as "statins," these medications lower cholesterol levels (LDL levels) by targeting triglycerides. They are used to treat patients with high cholesterol and coronary heart disease.

Types: Atorva**statin** (Lipitor), lova**statin** (Mevacor), rosuva**statin** (Crestor), simva**statin** (Zocor), prava**statin** (Pravachol), and fluva**statin** (Lescol). Other types of treatments are gemfibrozil (Lopid) and ezetimibe (Zetia) to treat high cholesterol.

Contraindications: Pregnant patients should use caution when taking these medications.

Pharmacokinetics: Metabolized by the liver.

Side Effects: Hepatotoxicity, myopathy, muscle cramps, headache, abdominal pain, muscle breakdown, and diarrhea.

Nursing Care: Monitor liver enzymes closely. Assess for muscle pain or weakness. Administer medications in the evening. Monitor cholesterol levels. Monitor patients who are on anticoagulants while on this medication.

Bile Acid Sequestrants

Definition: These medications are used to decrease cholesterol levels and triglycerides. They are typically used in conjunction with a statin.

Types: Cholestyramine (Questran) and colestipol (Colestid) are commonly used.

Contraindications: Patients who suffer from irritable bowel syndrome or GI issues should use caution when taking this medication.

Pharmacokinetics: Metabolized in the intestine and excreted through the feces.

Side Effects: Bloating, nausea, diarrhea, and GI upset.

Nursing Care: Bile acid sequestrants should be given with food or mixed in juice. The drug is a powdered substance that needs to be mixed. Bile acid sequestrants should be given 1 to 2 hours apart from other medications to avoid potential drug interactions. Teach the patient to monitor for any side effects.

Antiplatelet Medications

Definition: These medications are used to prevent the formation of plaque build-up and thrombus in the arteries. Blockage of the arteries can cause serious complications such as stroke or MI.

Types: Aspirin (ASA), triofiban (Aggrastat), clopidogrel (Plavix), ticlopidine (Ticlid), and cilostazol (Pletal).

Contraindications: Patients with bleeding disorders should stop taking antiplatelet medications. They are also instructed to stop all antiplatelet medications before surgeries or invasive procedures.

Pharmacokinetics: Metabolized and excreted by the liver.

→ *Side Effects:* **Bruising, GI bleeding, GI upset, anemia, dizziness, and headache.**

Nursing Care: Monitor for signs of bleeding. Teach the patient to assess for side effects. If the patient is experiencing dark stool or frank blood through the stool, stop all antiplatelet medications. Monitor liver functions. **The patient should take precautions against bleeding while on these medications, such as shaving with an electric razor, applying pressure to small cuts, avoiding bruises, and using a soft toothbrush.** As these medications can cause GI upset, they should be taken with food. Patients are instructed to stop these medications before any procedure. Patients who have cardiac surgery or blood clots are placed on long-term antiplatelet therapy.

Anticoagulants

Definition: Anticoagulants are used to dissolve blood clots and prevent further thrombosis by coagulating (thinning) the blood. They are used to treat patients with atrial fibrillation, and those at risk for or with deep vein thrombosis or pulmonary embolism (PE).

Types: **Heparin (IV, PO, or subQ), warfarin (Coumadin), enoxaparin (Lovenox), tinzaparin (Innohep), dalteparin (Fragmin), dabagatran (Pradaxa), and fondaparinux (Arixtra).**

Contraindications: Individuals with bleeding disorders should stop or use caution when taking these medications.

Pharmacokinetics: Metabolized and excreted by the liver.

Side Effects: **Easy bruising, hemorrhage, bleeding in the gums, GI bleed, and heparin-induced thrombocytopenia.**

Nursing Care: Coumadin is often used to treat blood clots, PE, and atrial fibrillation. Coumadin dosage is controlled and based on the individual's prothrombin time (PT) and international normalized ratio (INR) to clotting factors. **The normal PT level is 10 to 12 seconds and INR is 1.2 to 2.0. An INR less than 3 can mean the patient is at risk for bleeding and the dose may need to be stopped or decreased.** Patients are instructed to have the PT/INR checked frequently. Teach the patient about the side effects and risks of taking Coumadin. The medication is typically given at the same time every day. The antidote for Coumadin is vitamin K.

Heparin prevents clots by activating fibrinogen and fibrin. Heparin helps convert fibrinogen to fibrin to dissolve clots. Heparin is effective and based on an individual's partial prothrombin time (PTT). Now, here is a little trick, because you will be tested on the two main anticoagulants. **Heparin goes with PTT, and Coumadin goes with PT; now if you write out PTT and cross the two T's it creates an "H" to represent heparin.** Heparin can be given IV or subcutaneously. If a patient is admitted for a blood clot or a PE, a heparin drip is typically ordered, and the PTT is monitored every 6 hours until levels are therapeutic. Follow the heparin protocol at your facility. Monitor for signs of bleeding. The antidote for heparin is protamine sulfate.

Lovenox is similar to heparin but not as potent. Lovenox is given subcutaneously in the abdomen or arm. There are no clotting factors that need to be monitored with Lovenox. The injection site may cause severe bruising, so instruct the patient not to rub or apply pressure to the area after administering. Monitor for signs of bleeding. The antidote for Lovenox is protamine sulfate.

Thrombolytics

Definition: Thrombolytic medications are also used to dissolve blood clots by activating plasmin to break up clots. **They are used to treat patients with myocardial infarction, pulmonary embolism, DVTs, and stroke.**

Types: Altepl**ase** (Activase), tenectepl**ase** (TNKase), and streptokinase (Strepltase) are commonly given.

Contraindications: Patients with bleeding disorders should not use this medication.

Pharmacokinetics: Metabolized by the liver and excreted through the urine.

Side Effects: Bruising and bleeding.

Nursing Care: **Thrombolytic therapy has to meet the criteria of administering the medication to patients with MI and stroke within 3 hours of symptom onset**. Monitor clotting factors while patients are on these medications. Monitor for signs of bleeding. If medication therapy cannot be administered, surgical interventions may be needed. Place the patient on bleeding precautions. Closely monitor patients.

Cardiac Glycosides

Definition: These medications increase contractility and cardiac output. Cardiac glycosides also decrease sodium and potassium levels. They are used for patients with cardiac tachycardia and heart failure.

Types: Digoxin (Lanoxin).

Contraindicated: Caution should be used when administering to patients with renal failure or those with electrolyte imbalances.

Pharmacokinetics: Metabolized and excreted through the kidneys.

Side Effects: Visual disturbances, nausea, vomiting, weight loss, bradycardia, hypokalemia, dizziness, tachycardia, and fatigue.

Nursing Care: Before administering, take the apical pulse for a full minute. If the pulse is less than 60 bpm, hold the medication. This medication can decrease the pulse severely. **Complications such as digitalis toxicity can occur when taking this medication. Labs are obtained to monitor digoxin levels, which range from 0.5 to 2.0 ng/mL.** The signs of digoxin toxicity are nausea, vomiting, green halos, and cardiac dysrhythmias. The antidote for digoxin is digoxin immune fab (Digibind). If an irregular heartbeat or rhythm occurs while a patient is taking this medication, the drug should be stopped and the physician contacted immediately. Cardiac monitoring is ordered.

Vasodilators

Definition: Vasodilators work by dilating the blood vessels and increasing oxygen supply, especially in areas where ischemia is present. They are used to treat patients with angina, MI, or hypertension associated with chest discomfort.

Types: Nitroglycerin paste (Nitro-Bid), nitroglycerin sublingual (Nitrostat), isosorbide mononitrate (Imdur), isosorbide dinitrate (Isordil), and hydralazine (Apresoline) are used.

Contraindications: Patients who are hypotensive should not use these medications.

Pharmacokinetics: They are absorbed by the liver and excreted through the urine. Patients who take sildenafil (Viagra) should avoid nitrates due to the side effect of severe hypotension.

Side Effects: Hypotension, headache, reflex tachycardia, syncope, and dizziness.

Nursing Care: Monitor the patient's blood pressure and pulse before administering, paying attention to any parameters. Nitrates given sublingually should be taken while the patient is sitting down. Nitroglycerin tablets are kept in a dark bottle in a cool place. **Three tablets are given in 5-minute intervals, and if chest pain is not relieved by the third dose, a more aggressive treatment may be needed.**

Nitroglycerin ointment should be applied with gloves and dosed based on using a ruler-type paper. The dose is usually ½ or 1 inch of ointment. The paper is then placed on the right or left chest or back. Tape the piece of paper, but remove if any signs of hypotension occur. Gloves should always be worn, as touching the ointment with bare hands can cause fainting or dizziness.

Antiarrhythmic Medications

Definition: These medications control conduction of the heart and regulate the pattern or rhythm.

Types: Atropine (subQ or IV), adenosine (IV), amiodarone (PO or IV), quinidine sulfate (PO), or mexiletine (PO). Other medications, such as calcium channel blockers and beta-blockers, are used to treat irregular rhythms.

Contraindications: Patients with cardiac defects.

Pharmacokinetics: Metabolized by the liver and excreted through the urine.

Side Effects: Hypotension, dizziness, bradycardia, and edema.

→ *Nursing Care:* Monitor vital signs before administering. **These medications can be given in emergency situations to treat bradycardia and cardiac arrest.** Cardiac monitoring is ordered, and → these patients are commonly placed on a telemetry unit. **Intravenous medications should be given slowly over a 5-minute period, with frequent monitoring of vital signs.** Monitor electrolytes.

RESPIRATORY MEDICATIONS

Bronchodilators

Definition: Bronchodilators are used to dilate the bronchioles to reduce airway restriction and facilitate better breathing. There are two types: short-acting and long-acting inhalants. These medications are used to treat shortness of breath, COPD exacerbations, asthma, pneumonia, bronchitis, em- → physema, and bronchospasms. **Most medications that end in "-erol" are used to treat respiratory conditions.**

Types: Short-acting beta2-adrenergic agonists, short-acting anticholinergics, long-acting beta2-adrenergic agonists, and long-acting cholinergics.

I. Short-Acting Beta2-Adrenergic Agonists

Definition: Short-acting inhalants are used to treat a number of respiratory disorders. They are also known as *rescue inhalers* due to their rapid relief and onset. At times, this medication is used in conjunction with the anticholinergic ipratropium bromide (Atrovent) to facilitate better breathing.

Types: Albut**erol** (Proventil or Ventolin), levalbut**erol** (Xopenex), terbutaline (Brethine), pirbut**erol** (Maxair), and metaproterenol (Alupent).

Contraindications: Patients with tachycardia or cardiac dysrhythmias should not use these medications.

Pharmacokinetics: These medications are inhaled and have a 4- to 6-hour duration.

Side Effects: **Tachycardia, anxiety, tremors, nervousness, cough, headache, hyperglycemia, mouth dryness, and cardiac dysrhythmias.** ←

Nursing Care: **Assess the heart rate before administering medication, and listen to lung sounds.** Obtain an O_2 stat before and after treatment. Patients should avoid caffeinated beverages or other stimulants while taking this medication. Teach the patient the side effects of this medication. Smoking cessation is offered. An antianxiety medication may be needed to treat nervousness and anxiety. ←

II. Short-Acting Anticholinergics

Definition: These medications are used to smooth bronchial muscles to facilitate better breathing and decrease secretions. They are used to treat a wide array of respiratory disorders.

Types: Ipratropium (Atrovent), an aerosol.

Contraindications: Hypertension, children with diabetes, and those with a peanut allergy.

Pharmacokinetics: Inhalant with a duration of 4 to 6 hours.

Side Effects: **Dry mouth, cough, and nasal dryness.** ←

Nursing Care: Due to the side effect of dry mouth, instruct the patient to rinse with water after treatment. Monitor for side effects. If a long-acting anticholinergic is needed, tiotropium (Spiriva) is given.

III. Long-Acting Beta2-Adrenergic Agonists

Definition: Long-acting inhalants are used for bronchodilation and to decrease the inflammatory response in the lungs.

Types: Salmeterol (Serevent) and formoterol (Foradil).

Contraindications: Patients with diabetes and those with a history of cardiac dysrhythmias.

Pharmacokinetics: An inhalant with a long duration of 12 hours.

Side Effects: Hyperglycemia, tachycardia, bronchospasms, and dry mouth.

Nursing Care: Teach the patient the side effects of these medications, and continue to monitor HR, O_2, and lung sounds. **Magnesium infusions are used to treat bronchospasms.**

IV. Methylxanthines

Definition: These medications are used to treat nocturnal asthma symptoms and facilitate better breathing.

Types: Aminophylline (Phyllocontin)

Contraindication: Patients who take digoxin should use caution when taking this medication due to the risk of digoxin toxicity.

Pharmacokinetics: Metabolized by the liver and excreted through the urine.

Side Effects: Headache, GI upset, difficulty urinating, and dry mouth.

Nursing Care: Obtain vital signs before administrating, and assess lung sounds. This medication should be given on an empty stomach. Monitor for side effects.

Corticosteroids

Definition: Corticosteroids are inflammatory agents that decrease mucous production and promote relaxation of the bronchial muscles. They are often used in conjunction with bronchodilators. Corticosteroids are administered orally, intravenously, or inhaled.

Types: Inhalants are fluticasone (Flovent), triamcinolone acetonide (Azmacort), and beclomethasone (Beclovent). Oral corticosteroids are prednisone. Intravenous corticosteroid is methylprednisolone (Solu-Medrol).

Contraindications: Corticosteroids tend to increase blood glucose levels, and diabetic patients should use caution when taking.

Pharmacokinetics: Inhalant corticosteroids are absorbed by the lungs and are less effective than oral steroids.

Side Effects: **Thrush, Cushing's syndrome, hyperglycemia, edema, cough, nausea, vomiting, nervousness, acne, dry throat and mouth.**

Nursing Care: Corticosteroids do not provide fast-acting relief and may need to be used with albuterol to treat patients with asthma, COPD, or pneumonia. They are not used to treat acute symptoms. Patients should rinse the mouth after administration to avoid thrush. **Patients are instructed not to suddenly stop medication, but to slowly taper off of it.** Assess and treat side effects.

Leukotriene Modifiers

Definition: These medications decrease inflammation in the bronchioles and dilate smooth muscles in the respiratory tract. They are used for patients with chronic asthma and allergic rhinitis. They are given once a day in the evening. Take 1 hour before meals or 2 hours after.

Types: Montelukast (Singulair), zafirlukast (Accolate), and zileuton (Zyflo).

Contraindications: Patients with acute asthma or liver disease should not take these medications.

Pharmacokinetics: Leukotrine modifiers are absorbed by the lungs and bind to albumin. They are metabolized by the liver.

Side Effects: Headache, dry mouth, nausea, and dizziness.

Nursing Care: Monitor liver function tests (LFTs). Monitor side effects and treat as ordered.

Mucolytic Medications

Definition: Mucolytics break up mucus in the bronchial tubes, which is expelled through coughing. They are used for patients with chest congestion.

Types: Acetylcysteine (Mucomyst), guaifenesin (Mucinex, Robitussin).

Contraindications: Children younger than 12 years of age should not use this medication.

Pharmacokinetics: Excreted through the kidneys.

Side Effects: Moist cough, nausea, and GI upset.

Nursing Care: Mucomyst is administered through a nebulizer, and Mucinex is given orally. Assess for GI upset.

Antihistamines (H_1 Blockers)

Definition: These medications block H_1 receptors to decrease nasal congestion and dilate bronchial muscles. Antihistamines are used for patients who suffer from seasonal allergies and motion sickness.

Types: Diphenhydramine (Benadryl), loratadine (Claritin), cetrizine hydrocholoride (Zyrtec), desloratadine (Clarinex), and fexofenadine (Allegra). There are lots of antihistamines out there; these are only some of the common ones used.

Contraindications: Patients with kidney disorders.

Pharmacokinetics: Metabolized by the liver.

Side Effects: Drowsiness, hypotension, constipation, dry mouth, and GI upset.

→ *Nursing Care:* **Patients should use caution when taking these medications since they can cause drowsiness.** Take at bedtime. Assess for GI upset. They are also used for allergic reactions and pruritus.

Tuberculosis Medications

Definition: They are used to treat tuberculosis and decrease its transmission. **These medications are taken over a period of 6 to 9 months, and sputum cultures are monitored.** →

Types: There are two types of first-line and second-line treatments. They will be explained in detail below.

I. Isoniazid (INH)

Definition: First-line treatment for TB.

Side Effects: Night sweats, vision changes, cough, dry mouth, hyperglycemia, hepatitis, and hepatotoxicity.

Contraindication: Pregnant women and patients with liver disease.

Nursing Care: Monitor liver and renal function before administering medication. Teach the patient about the side effects and to assess signs of hepatotoxicity. Instruct the patient to take the medications on an empty stomach, with water, either 1 hour before meals or 2 hours after. Avoid foods with tyramine as they can cause a severe reaction with INH. Lab work is conducted frequently during treatment. The patient is placed on droplet precautions and placed in a negative-pressure room to avoid transmission to others.

II. Rifampin (Rifadin) or rifapentine (Priftin)

Definition: This first-line treatment inhibits RNA synthesis of TB bacillus.

→ *Side Effects:* **Red-orange secretions (sweat/urine), night sweats, bone pain, hepatotoxicity, hepatitis, and GI upset.**

Contraindication: Caution should be used when administering to pregnant women and patients with liver disease. Rifampin may also decrease the effectiveness of Coumadin.

Nursing Care: Monitor liver function and uric acid levels. Teach the patient about side effects and to watch for signs of hepatotoxicity. This medication should be taken on an empty stomach.

III. Pyrazinamide (PZA)

Definition: PZA is used in conjunction with other tuberculosis medications. PZA attacks the site of infection and decreases bacterial organisms.

Side Effects: **Hepatotoxicity, hepatitis, visual changes, and joint pain.** ←

Contraindication: Pregnant women and those with liver disorder.

Nursing Care: Assess uric acids and liver function tests. Instruct the patient to take with food to avoid GI upset.

IV. Ethambutol (Myambutol)

Definition: This medication treats TB by attacking the site of infection.

Side Effects: Dizziness, nausea, vomiting, increased uric acid, joint pain, hepatotoxicity, rash, and **vision changes.** ←

Contraindication: Children should not take this medication due to the side effects.

Nursing Care: Assess for vision changes or dizziness. Provide safety measures if patient's gait is affected. Take medications with food to decrease GI upset.

NEUROLOGICAL MEDICATIONS

Thrombolytics: Most "-ase" Endings

Definition: They dissolve clots by increasing plasminogen, which activates plasmin to help break up or dissolve clots. Alteplase is used for patients who suffer ischemic strokes or MI.

Types: **Alteplase (Activase), tenecteplase (TNKase), and streptase are commonly given.** ←

Contraindications: Patients with bleeding disorders should not use this medication.

Pharmacokinetics: Metabolized by the liver and excreted through the urine.

Side Effects: Bruising and bleeding.

Nursing Care: **Thrombolytic therapy has to meet the criteria of administering the medication to patients with MI and stroke within 3 hours of symptom onset.** ← Do not give these medications to patients with hemorrhagic bleeds. Monitor clotting factors while patients are on these medications. Monitor for signs of bleeding. If medication therapy cannot be administered, surgical interventions may be needed. Place patient on bleeding precautions. Closely monitor patients. **Monitor labs PT, INR, platelets, and PTT.** ←

Treatment of Increased Intracranial Pressure

Definition: Osmotic diuretics decrease reabsorption of water and electrolytes. Mannitol is used to treat patients with increased ICP.

→ *Types:* **Mannitol (Osmitrol)**

Contraindication: Patients who are in renal failure.

Pharmacokinetics: Given intravenously and excreted through the urine.

Side Effects: Headache, GI upset, edema, orthostatic hypotension, and electrolyte imbalance.

Nursing Care: Monitor vital signs, mental status, labs, and urine output. Conduct neurological checks every 2 to 4 hours. Patients are kept on bed rest, and a Foley catheter is usually placed. → **Patients may also be in an induced coma until there is a decrease in ICP.** If the mannitol vial contains crystals, discard the vial and obtain another vial.

Antiepileptic Medications

Definition: Seizures cause abnormal firing of neurons in the brain, and antiepileptic medications work to control and decrease this firing to control seizures. They are used to treat grand mal and focal seizures.

Types: phenobarbital (Sodium Luminal), primidone (Mysoline), clonazepam (Klonopin), carbamazepine (Tegretol), phenytoin (Dilantin), fosphenytoin (Cerebyx), valproic acid (Depakote), lamotrigine (Lamictal), ethosuximide (Zarontin), oxcarbazepin (Trileptal), and levetiracetam (Keppra).

Contraindications: Patients taking oral contraceptives, anticoagulants, and benzodiazepines should use caution when taking these medications. Patients with liver disease should use caution when taking these medications.

Pharmacokinetics: Can be given IV or PO. Metabolized by the liver and excreted through the urine.

→ *Side Effects:* **Double vision, drowsiness, unsteady gait, bradycardia, confusion, headache, gingival hyperplasia, fatigue, nausea, vomiting, rash, and cardiac dysrhythmias.**

Nursing Care: Monitor vital signs and have a baseline neurological examination performed. Place the patient on seizure precautions. Assess for side effects such as vision changes and ensure good oral care to avoid gingival hyperplasia. Intravenous medications are given only in the hospital; medications such as oral Keppra are given to control and prevent seizures. Instruct the patient never to stop these medications abruptly. Monitor liver function tests.

Medications for Parkinson's Disease

I. Dopaminergic Medications

Definition: These are dopaminergic drugs that treat symptoms associated with Parkinson's disease by decreasing acetylcholine and increasing dopamine.

Types: Levodopa (L-DOPA), and carbidopa-levodopa (Sinemet)

Contraindication: Patients taking monoamine oxidase inhibitors should use caution when taking these medications.

Pharmacokinetics: Taken orally, metabolized by the liver, and excreted through the urine.

Side Effects: **Urinary retention, dry mouth, GI upset, dyskinesia, and hypotension.** ←

Nursing Care: Monitor vital signs, neurological status, and urinary output. Assess and teach the patient the side effects of this medication. The patient should avoid alcohol while taking this this medication. Do not stop this medication abruptly as it needs to be tapered off.

II. Dopamine Agonists

Definition: Dopamine agonists work to activate dopamine receptors to treat and decrease symptoms associated with Parkinson's disease.

Types: Ropinirole (Requip), bromocriptine (Parlodel), pramipexole (Mirapex), amantadine (Symmetrel), rasagline (Azilect), and apomorphine (Apokyn).

Contraindications: Patients with kidney failure and liver disease should use caution.

Pharmacokinetics: Taken orally, metabolized by the liver, and excreted through the urine.

Side Effects: GI upset, dizziness, sleepiness, hypotension, dyskinesia, hallucinations, and constipation.

Nursing Care: Administer medications with food to avoid GI upset. These medications work over time to decrease symptoms associated with Parkinson's disease. Teach the patient to assess side effects and report any changes to the physician. Use caution when driving due to dizziness.

Medications for Myasthenia Gravis/Cholinergic Medications

Definition: These medications work to increase the mimic acetylcholine's CNS effect and increase its levels in the body.

Types: neostig**mine** (Prostigmin), pyridostig**mine** (Mestinon), rivastig**mine** (Exelon), and ambenoium (Mytelase).

Contraindication: Patients taking antihistamines, antidepressants, and antipsychotics should use caution when taking these medications.

Pharmacokinetics: Given PO, IV, or IM and excreted through the urine.

Side Effects: Bradycardia, GI upset, sweating, excessive salivation, wheezing, and urinary urgency.

→ *Nursing Care:* Administer medications 30 minutes before a meal. Obtain vital signs before administering medication. Assess for the complication of cholinergic crisis. **Mestinon is used to continuously treat myasthenia gravis, and edrophonium (Tensilon) is used to diagnose it. Atropine is used as an antidote. Continue to monitor for side effects.**

Medications for Multiple Sclerosis

Definition: Immunomodulators are administered to help regulate the immune system and are often given to multiple sclerosis patients. Immunomodulators decrease destruction of myelin in order to suppress symptoms of multiple sclerosis.

Types: Interferon beta-1a (Avonex and Rebif) and glatiramer acetate (Copaxone).

Contraindication: Patients with liver disease should use caution when taking these medications.

Pharmacokinetics: Given through injection subcutaneously. Metabolized by the liver and excreted through the urine.

Side Effects: Headache, pain, cough, muscle aches, and fever.

→ *Nursing Care:* **Assess liver function tests before starting medication.** Teach and assess for side effects. Flulike symptoms are common with these medications. The injection site may be sore, as well.

ENDOCRINE MEDICATIONS

Medications for Patients With Diabetes

I. Oral Hypoglycemic Medications

Definition: These medications stimulate beta cells to increase insulin production in the pancreas. They are used to treat patients with diabetes mellitus type 2.

Types:

- **Sulfonylureas**: Glipizide (Glucotrol), glyburide (Micronase), tolbutamide (Orinase), gliclazide (Diamicron), tolazamide (Tolinase), and glimepiride (Amaryl).
- **Meglitinides:** Repaglinide (Prandin) and nateglinide (Starlix).
- **Biguanides**: Metformin (Glucophage)
- **Thiazolidinediones:** Rosiglitazone (Avandia) and pioglitazone (Actos)
- **Dipeptidyl Peptidase-4 Inhibitors**: Stigaliptin phosphate (Januvia) and vildagliptin (Galvus).
- **Alpha-Glucosidase Inhibitors**: Acarbose (Precose) and miglitol (Glyset)

Contraindications: Patients with kidney, liver, or heart failure should not use these medications.

Pharmacokinetics: Taken orally, metabolized by the liver, and excreted through the urine.

Side Effects: Hypoglycemia, GI upset, rash, nausea, metallic taste in mouth, dizziness, weight gain, edema, and diarrhea.

Nursing Care: Obtain blood glucose levels and hemoglobin A1C levels. **These medications are typically given with breakfast or dinner. Monitor side effects and hypoglycemia. If blood glucose is less than 70, or if a patient has poor PO intake, hold PO hypoglycemic medications.** Other medications such as beta-adrenergic blockers can mask signs of hypoglycemia, and corticosteroids can increase blood glucose levels. Monitor for weight gain and edema.

II. Insulin

Definition: Insulin is injected into fat and muscles to decrease overall glucose levels. It causes the liver, fat tissue, and muscles to absorb glucose and used to treat patients with diabetes mellitus types 1 and 2.

Types of Insulin:

- Rapid-acting insulin has an onset of 15 minutes, peaks in 60 to 90 minutes, and has a duration of 3 to 4 hours. Types are lispro (Humalog), insulin aspart (Novolog), and insulin glulisine (Apidra).
- Short-acting insulin has an onset of 30 minutes to 1 hour, peaks in 2 to 3 hours, and lasts 3 to 6 hours. Regular insulin (Novolin R and Humulin R) is short-acting insulin.
- Intermediate insulin has an onset of 2 to 4 hours, peaks in 4 to 10 hours, and lasts for 10 to 16 hours. Types are neutral protamine Hagedron (NPH) Humulin N, or Novolin N. Can be mixed with regular insulin.

- Long-acting insulin has an onset of 1 to 2 hours, no peak, and lasts for 24 hours. Types are glargine (Lantus) and detemir (Levemir).

Contraindication: Patients with renal failure and hypoglycemic patients should use caution when taking insulin.

Pharmacokinetics: Taken subcutaneously, metabolized by the pancreas, and excreted through the urine.

Side Effects: Hypoglycemia.

Nursing Care: Obtain glucose level before administering insulin. An insulin sliding scale is used to dose the amount of insulin that is required. If a patient is NPO or has poor PO intake, insulin may be held. → **Infections, surgery, and corticosteroids can increase glucose levels**. Patients are placed on a diabetic diet. Insulin is administered subcutaneously in the arm, thigh, or abdomen; rotate site with each administration. Patients who take long-acting insulin are typically given Lantus at night before bedtime. → **NPH and regular insulin are mixed at times. Remember, clear before cloudy when mixing. NPH is cloudy, and regular insulin is clear.** Teach the patient to monitor for signs of hypoglycemia. Hypoglycemia can cause severe weakness, syncope, sweating, and flushed appearance. Treatment is giving two cups of orange juice or graham crackers, or administering D5 to the patient. Frequently assess blood glucose levels. Diet and exercise can help decrease blood glucose levels.

Adrenocortical Medications

I. Corticosteroids

Definition: These medications decrease systemic inflammation.

Types: Prednisone (Orasone), IV methylprednisolone sodium succinate (Solu-Medrol), dexamethasone (Decadron), and hydrocortisone (Solu-Cortef).

Contraindications: Patients with renal failure, immunosuppressed, or diabetes should use these medications with caution.

Pharmacokinetics: Can be given orally or intravenously; works systemically to decrease inflammation.

→ *Side Effects:* **Hyperglycemia, weight gain, skin thinning (prednisone skin), osteoporosis, GI upset, bruising, hypokalemia, slow wound healing, and hyponatremia.**

Nursing Care: Assess renal function, glucose, and weight before administration. Monitor for side effects and treat as ordered. Glucose levels increase with medications and may need to be treated with insulin in the hospital. Patients who are on long-term antibiotics have slow wound healing and thinning of the skin. Patients are prone to skin tears and bruises. Proper skin care and caution need to be in place.

II. Mineralocorticoids

Definition: These medications are **used to treat Addison's disease. Mineralocorticoids help by increasing aldosterone to maintain electrolyte balance.** ←

Types: Fludrocortisone acetate (Florinef Acetate)

Contraindications: Patients with renal and heart failure should use caution when taking these medications.

Pharmacokinetics: Metabolized by the kidneys and excreted through the urine.

Side Effects: Electrolyte imbalance (hypokalemia, hyponatremia, and hypocalcemia), weight gain, edema, and bone loss.

Nursing Care: Monitor electrolytes before administering medication. Report any bone pain or cramping to the physician. Calcium, potassium, and sodium supplements may need to be given. Monitor patients for cardiac palpitations. Give medications with food. **Daily weights should be obtained as well to monitor edema and weight gain.** ←

III. Adrenal Corticosteroid Inhibitors

Definition: These medications decrease hormone production of the adrenal glands. They are used to treat Cushing's syndrome.

Types: Aminoglutethimide (Cytadren) and metyrapone (Metopirone)

Contraindications: Patients with shingles or chicken pox should not take these medications, and those with renal failure should use caution when taking them.

Pharmacokinetics: These medications are metabolized by the liver and excreted through the urine.

Side Effects: Dizziness, headache, loss of appetite, nausea, weakness, and severe allergic reaction can occur.

Nursing Care: Teach the patient the side effects of the medication. Give medication with food to decrease GI upset. Assess for signs of improvement in Cushing's syndrome.

Medications for Hypothyroidism

Definition: These medications are used to increase and stimulate levels of thyroxine and triiodothyronine (T3 and T4) to help maintain healthy thyroid function.

Types: Levothyroxine (Levothyroid, Levoxyl, or Synthroid), dessicated thyroid extract (Armour Thyroid), liotrix (Thyrolar), and liothyronine sodium (Cytomel).

Contraindications: Many drug interactions can occur with this medication. **Patients taking Coumadin or Dilantin may benefit from these medications as they can increase effectiveness.**

Pharmacokinetics: Metabolized by the liver and excreted by the urine.

Side Effects: **Sweating, chest pain, tachycardia, heat intolerance, abdominal cramps, decreased appetite, nervousness, insomnia, esophageal atresia, and hyperthyroidism can occur.**

Nursing Care: Monitor thyroid levels, vital signs, and daily weight. Thyroid medications are taken 1 to 2 hours before a meal in the morning and given with a full glass of water. Monitor for side effects.

Medications for Hyperthyroidism

Definition: These medications are used to decrease thyroid hormone levels in patients with hyperthyroidism and Graves' disease.

Types: **Methimazole (Tapazole), radioactive iodine, potassium chloride (Lugol's solution).**

Contraindication: Pregnant women should use caution when taking these medications because of the iodine content.

Pharmacokinetics: Metabolized by the liver and excreted through the urine.

Side Effects: Headache, GI upset, dizziness, agranulocytosis, and iodine toxicity. Signs of iodine toxicity are brassy taste, headache, gum erosion, and abdominal pain.

Nursing Care: Monitor thyroid levels, vital signs, and daily weight. Monitor for signs of iodine toxicity. These medications are given in the morning before breakfast.

Medications for Hyperparathyroidism

Definition: These medications are used to prevent the loss of calcium in the bones. They decrease calcium levels produced by the parathyroid gland.

Types: Bisphosphonates such as alendronate (Fosamax), risedronate sodium (Actonel), calcitonin-salmon (Miacalcin), ibandronate (Boniva), etidronate (Didronel), and pamidronate

(Aredia). Calcimimetics such as cinacalcet (Sensipar) are also used.

Contraindications: Patients with osteoporosis and renal failure should use caution when taking these medications.

Pharmacokinetics: Metabolized by the liver and excreted through the urine. Can be given orally, subcutaneously, or intranasally.

Side Effects: Headache, GI upset, tetany, skeletal pain, and blurred vision.

Nursing Care: **Monitor calcium levels. Fosamax should be taken with a full glass of water and the patient should sit upright for an hour after administration to avoid GI upset.** ←

Medications for Hypoparathyroidism

Definition: Calcium supplements are given to increase calcium levels.

Types: Calcium carbonate (Os-Cal, TUMS, Rolaids, or Caltrate), calcium acetate (PhosLo), calcium citrate (Citracal), and calcium gluconate are commonly given.

Contraindication: Patients with kidney failure should use caution when taking these medications.

Pharmacokinetics: Can be given orally or intravenously. Absorbed through the bones and excreted through the urine.

Side Effects: GI upset, constipation, fractures, and cardiac arrhythmias.

Nursing Care: **Monitor calcium levels. Due to loss of calcium, bone loss can occur, putting the patient at risk for fractures. Cardiac monitoring may be needed.** ←

Pancreatic Enzymes

Definition: These medications are used to replace enzymes that help with digestion.

Types: Pancreatin (Creon) and pancrelipase (Pancrease)

Contraindication: Patients with liver and renal failure should use caution when taking these medications.

Pharmacokinetics: Metabolized by the liver and excreted through the urine.

Side Effects: GI upset.

Nursing Care: **Given 1 hour after meals and should never be crushed. Can also be used to increase appetite.** ←

GASTROINTESTINAL MEDICATIONS

Histamine 2-Receptor Antagonists (H_2 Blockers): All "-idine" Endings

Definition: These block H_2 receptors to decrease acid in the stomach. They are used for patients with peptic ulcer disease and GERD.

Types: Raniti**dine** (Zantac), cimeti**dine** (Tagamet), nizati**dine** (Axid), and famoti**dine** (Pepcid).

Contraindication: Patients with liver or kidney disease should use caution when taking these medications. Patients on Coumadin or Dilantin should not take Tagamet.

Pharmacokinetics: Metabolized by the liver and excreted through the urine. Tagamet crosses the blood-brain barrier and causes CNS effects. H_2 blockers can be given PO, IV, or IM.

Side Effects: Confusion, hallucinations, cardiac dysthymias, and anxiety.

→ *Nursing Care:* These medications **should be taken 30 minutes before or after a meal. Tagamet should be taken with food, and oral antacids should be avoided. Zantac should not be taken with aspirin. Give 1 hour after antacids. Use caution when combining with NSAIDs.** Monitor for side effects. Pepcid can be given IV, but must be mixed with a 50 mL bag and hung over 15 to 30 minutes.

Proton Pump Inhibitors: All "-azole" Endings

Definition: Proton pump inhibitors inhibit gastric enzymes, thus decreasing acid production. They are used to treat peptic ulcer disease, GERD, and duodenal ulcers.

Types: Pantopr**azole** (Protonix), omepr**azole** (Prilosec), esomepr**azole** (Nexium), and lansopr**azole** (Prevacid).

Contraindications: Patients with gastric ulcers should use caution when taking these medications.

Pharmacokinetics: Metabolized by the liver and excreted by the urine.

Side Effects: Nausea, headache, dizziness, abdominal pain, bone loss, magnesium depletion, and hypertension.

Nursing Care: Advise the patient to take this medication 1 hour before meals and in the morning. Protonix can be given IV over 2 minutes and dilated in a 10 mL syringe. Monitor for side effects. → **Never crush or chew these medications.**

Antacids

Definition: Antacids decrease and neutralize gastric acid. They are used to treat GERD, ulcers, and peptic ulcer disease.

Types: Calcium carbonate (TUMS), magnesium hydroxide (Maalox, Milk of Magnesia), and aluminum hydroxide (Alu-Cap).

Contraindications: Patients with severe ulcer disease and renal disease should use caution when taking these medications. GI symptoms can sometimes signify cardiac problems. Assess both before administering these medications.

Pharmacokinetics: Metabolized by the liver and excreted through the urine.

Side Effects: Constipation, nausea, indigestion, electrolyte imbalance, and weight loss.

Nursing Care: **Instruct patients to take medications with a full glass of water and before meals or bedtime. Take 1 hour apart from other medications.** ←

Cytoprotective Agents

Definition: Cytoprotective agents decrease gastric acid and provide a protective coating in the stomach.

Types: Sucralfate (Carafate) and misoprostol (Cytotec).

Contraindications: Pregnant women should not use these medications.

Pharmacokinetics: Metabolized by the liver and excreted through the urine.

Side Effects: Abdominal pain, diarrhea, and constipation.

Nursing Care: **Carafate and cytotec should be given 30 minutes apart from antacids. Cytotec should be given with food, and carafate on an empty stomach. Instruct patients to avoid NSAIDs when using these medications.** ←

5 Aminosalicylates (5 ASA)

Definition: ASAs have anti-inflammatory effects in the small bowel and colon. They are used to treat ulcerative colitis and Crohn's disease.

Types: Sulfasalazine (Azulfidine) and mesalamine (Asacol, Pentasa).

Contraindications: Do not administer if patient has an allergy to sulfur products.

Pharmacokinetics: Absorbed by the small bowel and excreted through the urine.

Side Effects: Nausea, fatigue, fever, and rash.

Nursing Care: Maintain hydration, and monitor lab work such as a CBC. Monitor for side effects. Do not administer with diuretics.

Antiemetic Medications

I. Dopamine Antagonists

Definition: Block dopamine receptors to decrease feelings of nausea or vomiting.

Types: Prochlorperazine (Compazine), promethazine (Phenergan), metoclopramide (Reglan), or chlorpromazine (Thorazine).

Contraindication: Do not use with children. Patients with liver or kidney disease should use caution when taking these medications.

Pharmacokinetics: Given orally, IV, or IM. Metabolized by the liver and excreted through the urine or feces.

Side Effects: Dizziness, drowsiness, blurred vision, hypotension, and headache.

Nursing Care: Administer medication slowly. Monitor and teach the patient side effects. Phenergan can make patients very drowsy. → **Thorazine can be given to relieve hiccups.**

II. Serotonin Blockers: all "-setron" endings

Definition: Block serotonin (5-HT) receptors to decrease nausea and vomiting.

Types: Ondan**setron** (Zofran), dola**setron** (Anzemet), and grani**setron.**

Contraindications: Use with caution with patients with liver disease.

Pharmacokinetics: Metabolized by the liver and excreted through the urine. Can be given IV or PO.

Side Effects: Headache, rash, and diarrhea.

Nursing Care: Monitor for side effects.

Stool Softeners/Laxatives

Definition: Used to increase peristalsis to promote bowel movements and to treat constipation. There are many types of stool softeners and laxatives.

Types: Docusate sodium (Colace), sennosides (Sennakot/Senna), bisacodyl (Dulcolax), polyethylene glycol (GoLYTELY), magnesium hydroxide (Milk of Magnesia), sodium phosphate (Fleet enema), and psyllium (Metamucil).

Contraindications: Patients with bowel obstructions, ulcers, or diarrhea should not use these medications.

Pharmacokinetics: Metabolized by the intestines and excreted through the stool.

Side Effects: Electrolyte imbalance and diarrhea.

Nursing Care: Stool softeners should be given only temporarily until regular bowel movements occur. Laxatives should be taken only in severe cases of constipation. Pain medication can constipate patients, and a stool softener should be given in conjunction. Do not administer if patients are experiencing diarrhea or have *C. diff.* If the patient is experiencing diarrhea, monitor electrolytes. Increase fluid intake when taking these medications. **Patients taking GoLYTELY typically take it the night before in preparation for a colonoscopy.** Monitor for side effects. ←

Antidiarrheal Medications

Definition: Used to decrease peristalsis to help decrease bowel movements.

Types: Diphenoxylate/atropine (Lomotil) and loperamide (Imodium)

Contraindications: Pregnant women and those with GI bleeding should not take these medications.

Pharmacokinetics: Metabolized by the intestine and excreted through the stool.

Side Effects: Constipation.

Nursing Care: Monitor for constipation. Make sure patient is having regular bowel movements.

GENITOURINARY MEDICATIONS

Bladder Anticholinergics

Definition: These medications relax the bladder and decrease urinary output. They are used for patients with bladder spasms and overactive bladder.

Types: Oxybutynin (Ditropan), tolterodine (Detrol), and solifenacin succinate (Vesicare).

Contraindication: Patients with renal failure, urinary obstructions, or renal mass should use caution when taking these medications.

Pharmacokinetics: Metabolized by the kidneys and excreted through the urine.

Side Effects: GI upset, headache, dry mouth, tachycardia, urinary retention, and weakness.

Nursing Care: Monitor intake and output. Monitor for urinary retention. As most patients complain of dry mouth, increase fluid intake. To relieve symptoms of dry eyes, use eye drops.

Bladder Cholinergics (Muscarinic Agonists)

Definition: Bladder cholingerics contract the bladder and help empty it. They increase urinary output, and are used for patients with urinary retention not caused by an obstruction.

Types: Bethanecol chloride (Urecholine).

Contraindications: Patients with urinary obstructions should not take this medication. Patients with ulcers are not advised to take this medication.

Pharmacokinetics: Taken orally, metabolized by the kidneys, and excreted through the urine.

→ *Side Effects:* **Hypotension, nausea, vomiting, bradycardia, increased urine output, and bronchospasms.**

Nursing Care: This medication will increase urine output. Monitor output. This medication is taken in the morning on
→ an empty stomach. **A cholinergic crisis can occur whose symptoms are hypotension, bradycardia, and sweating. The antidote is atropine sulfate.**

Urinary Tract Antiseptics

Definition: These medications are used decrease and prevent the growth of bacteria that cause urinary tract infections.

Types: Nitrofurantoin (Furadantin/Macrobid), sulfamethoxale, and trimethoprim (Bactrim/Septra).

Contraindications: Patient with renal insufficiency should use caution with these medications.

Pharmacokinetics: Taken PO or IV, metabolized by the liver, and excreted by the kidneys.

→ *Side Effects:* GI upset, headache, depression, and **Stevens–Johnson syndrome.**

Nursing Care: Monitor renal function before starting medications. The patient's urine may be orange/brown in color. Give medications with a full glass of water or food. Assess for a sulfur allergy.

Urinary Analgesics

Definition: These medications are used to treat pain or burning related to urinary tract infections or bladder disorders.

Types: Phenazopyridine hydrochloride (Pyridium).

Contraindication: Patients with renal disease should not use these medications.

Pharmacokinetics: Metabolized by the kidneys and excreted through the urine.

Side Effects: Headache and GI upset.

Nursing Care: Can cause urine to turn orange, and stain clothing; relieves symptoms of burning when urinating.

Post-Transplant Immunosuppressants

Definition: These medications are used to decrease the body's immune response and help prevent rejection of transplanted organs (most often the kidney). There are many types, but I will discuss the most commonly given. Review the others in your textbook.

Types: Tacrolimus (Prograf), cyclosporine (Sandimmune), sirolimus (Rapamune), and mycophenolate mofetil (CellCept).

Contraindications: Patients with liver and renal failure should use caution when taking these medications.

Pharmacokinetics: Metabolized by the liver and excreted by the kidneys.

Side Effects: **Nephrotoxicity, hepatotoxicity, tremors, gingival hyperplasia, hypertension, seizures, and GI upset.** ←

Nursing Care: Monitor liver and renal function before administering these medications. Monitor blood pressure closely. Also monitor for infection, and for side effects, and report any changes to the physician.

MUSCULOSKELETAL MEDICATIONS

Medications to Treat Gout

Definition: These medications decrease uric acid production to reduce the symptoms of gout.

Types: Colchicine, allopurinol (Zyloprim), and probenecid (Benemid).

Contraindications: Patients with renal or cardiac disease should use caution when taking these medications.

Pharmacokinetics: Given orally, absorbed by the intestines, and excreted through the stool.

→ *Side Effects:* GI upset, kidney stones, and **bone marrow suppression.**

→ *Nursing Care:* **Monitor uric acid levels.** Take medications with food. Decrease purine in the diet. Elevate extremity if swollen.

Medications for Rheumatoid Arthritis

Definition: These medications decrease inflammation to relieve symptoms of rheumatoid arthritis.

Types: Nonsteroidal anti-inflammatory drugs (NSAIDs) are first-line treatment. Disease-modifying antirheumatic drugs (DMARDs) are used for second-line treatment. DMARDs are methotrexate (Rheumatrex), etanercept (Enbrel), adalimumab (Humira), hydroxychloroquine (Plaquenil), leflunimide (Arava), infliximab (Remicade), and abaracept (Orencia).

Contraindications: Patients with liver disease should use caution when taking these medications. Pregnant women should also avoid these medications.

Pharmacokinetics: Given orally or subcutaneously; metabolized by the liver and excreted through the urine.

Side Effects: Dizziness, headache, retinopathy, GI upset, fever, and chills.

Nursing Care: Monitor renal and liver function before administering. Give medications with food. Monitor side effects.

Treatment for Patients With Osteoporosis

Definition: These medications increase calcium in the bones.

Types: Alendro**nate** (Fosamax), ibandro**nate** (Boniva), raloxifene (Evista), and calcitonin-salmon (Calcimar).

Contraindications: Patients with hypercalcemia and esophagitis are instructed to use caution with these medications.

Pharmacokinetics: Give PO, intranasally, and IV. These medications are absorbed by the bones and metabolized by the kidneys.

Side Effects: **GI upset, esophagitis, rash, jaw pain, blurred vision, and fever.** ←

Nursing Care: Give medications on an empty stomach with a full glass of water, and wait 30 minutes to ensure absorption. Give medications with vitamin D. Monitor for skeletal pain.

Medications for Muscle Spasms

Definition: These medications relax skeletal muscle and decrease spasms by affecting the CNS system. They are used for patients who have chronic back pain and orthopedic surgery.

Types: Baclofen (Lioresal), tizanidine (Zanaflex), methocarbamol (Robaxin), cyclobenzaprine (Flexeril), carisoprodol (Soma), metaxalone (Skelaxin), diazepam (Valium), dantrolene (Dantrium).

Contraindication: Patients with liver or renal disease should use caution when taking these medications.

Pharmacokinetics: Taken PO, IV, or IM. These medications are metabolized by the liver and excreted through the urine.

Side Effects: Dizziness, drowsiness, fatigue, weakness, hypotension, visual changes, GI upset, and liver toxicity.

Nursing Care: Monitor mental status when administering medication as it can cause drowsiness and dizziness. Monitor blood pressure. Administer with meals. Instruct patients to avoid alcohol or opioids when taking this medication.

INTEGUMENTARY MEDICATIONS

Antifungals

Definition: These medications decrease fungal production at the cellular level. They are used for skin fungal infections.

Types: Clotrimazole (Lotrimin), terbinafine (Lamisil), ketoconazole (Nizoral), and nystatin (Mycolog).

Contraindications: Patients with liver problems should not use this medication.

Pharmacokinetics: Oral or topical. Metabolized by the liver and excreted by the kidneys.

Side Effects: Nausea, vomiting, rash, and abdominal pain.

Nursing Care: Apply to skin on infected areas, and assess for reaction of cream. They are not for long-term use.

Medications for Burns

Definition: These medications prevent and treat infection or burns.

Types: Silver nitrate, nitrofurazone (Furacin), silver sulfadiazine (Silvadene), and mafenide acetate (Sulfamylon 10%).

Contraindications: Patients with renal disease should use caution when taking these medications.

Pharmacokinetics: Absorbed by the skin and excreted through the kidneys.

Side Effects: Pain, burning, increased sensitivity, and rash.

Nursing Care: Spread a thin layer of Silvadene to the burn area. Monitor for pain and burning. Monitor renal function.

IMMUNOLOGICAL MEDICATIONS

Antiretroviral Medications

Definition: Antiretroviral therapy (ART) is used to treat patients with HIV/AIDS to suppress viral DNA and HIV transcriptase.

Types:

I. Nonnucleoside Reverse Transcriptase Inhibitors

Definition: These medications block the actions of reverse transcriptase, preventing HIV cells from converting RNA to DNA. They represent first-line treatment for HIV patients.

Types: Efavirenz (Sustive), delavirdine (Rescriptor), and nevirapine (Viramune).

Contraindications: Patients with liver disease should use caution with these medications.

Pharmacokinetics: Taken PO; they bind to protein and are excreted through the urine or stool.

→ *Side Effects:* **Rash, hepatotoxicity, GI upset, headache, dizziness, nightmares, and insomnia.**

Nursing Care: Monitor liver function tests and CD4 count. Instruct patients to take these medications in the morning on an empty stomach.

II. Nucleoside Reverse Transcriptase Inhibitors

Definition: These medications also block reverse transcriptase and decrease HIV replication.

Types: Abacavir (Ziagen), lamivudine (Epivir), didanosine (Videx), stavudine (Zerit), zidovudine (Retrovir), zalcitabine tenofovir (Viread), and emtricitabine (Emtriva).

Contraindications: Patients with liver or renal disease should not take these medications.

Pharmacokinetics: Taken orally, metabolized by the liver, and excreted through the urine.

Side Effects: **GI upset, bone marrow suppression, lactic acidosis, headache, fever, peripheral neuropathy, anemia, nausea, vomiting, and diarrhea.** ←

Nursing Care: Instruct patients to take on an empty stomach, and sit up for 30 minutes after administration. Monitor for side effects, and medicate as ordered. Instruct patients to avoid alcohol when taking these medications. Monitor liver functions and CD4 count.

III. Protease Inhibitors

Definition: These medications activate receptors to decrease HIV replication.

Types: Saquinavir (Fortovase), amprenavir (Agenerase), lopinavir/ritonavir (Kaletra), indinavir (Crixivan), nelfinavir (Viracept), ritonavir (Norvir), atazanavir (Reyataz), and fosamprenavir (Lexiva).

Contraindications: Patients with liver or renal disease should use caution when taking these medications.

Pharmacokinetics: Taken orally; metabolized by the liver and excreted through the urine.

Side Effects: GI upset, lipodystrophy, hyperlipidemia, drowsiness, headache, and fatigue.

Nursing Care: Monitor liver and renal function. Monitor CD4 count. Teach the patient about the side effects of the medication, and emphasize the importance of taking the medications daily. Patients with HIV/AIDS are immunocompromised and are susceptible to infections. Instruct patient to take medication on an empty stomach.

Chemotherapy

I. Alkylating Agents

Definition: These medications kill cells by alkylating the DNA.

Types: Cyclophosphamide (Cytoxan), busulfan (Myleran), ifosfamide (Ifex), mechlorethamine (Mustargen), carmustine (BiCNU), and chlorambucil (Leukeran).

Contraindications: Patients with renal disorders should use caution when taking these medications.

Pharmacokinetics: Given IV; crosses the blood-brain barrier, and is excreted through the urine.

→ *Side Effects:* **Hepatotoxicity, pulmonary infiltrates, cystitis, thrush, and bone marrow suppression.**

Nursing Care: Given IV through a port or IV. Monitor vital signs, respiratory status, and renal function. Monitor labs due to bone marrow suppression. Provide mouth care to avoid infection and thrush. Assess for a reaction to the chemotherapy.

II. Platinum Anticancer Medications

Definition: These medications are used to treat small cell lung carcinoma, ovarian cancer, lymphomas, and bladder, testicular, and cervical cancers.

Types: Cisplatin (Platinol) and carboplatin (Paraplatin)

Contraindications: Patients with liver and renal disease should use caution when taking these medications.

Pharmacokinetics: Given IV; crosses the blood-brain barrier, and is excreted through the urine.

→ *Side effects:* **Bone marrow suppression, neurotoxicity, ototoxicity, nausea, vomiting, hearing loss, fatigue, and alopecia.**

Nursing Care: Given IV through a port or IV line. Monitor vital signs, respiratory status, and renal function. Monitor labs due to bone marrow suppression. Provide mouth care to avoid infection and thrush. Assess for a reaction to the chemotherapy. → **Monitor for hearing loss.**

III. Antimetabolites

Definition: These medications inhibit cellular metabolism and disrupt nucleic acid function.

Types: Methotrexate sodium (Folex), pemetrexed (Alimta), cytarabine (Ara-C), capecitabine (Xeloda), fluorouracil (Adrucil), thioguanine (Tabloid), mercaptopurine (Purinethol), and gemcitabine (Gemzar).

Contraindication: Patients with liver or renal disease should use caution when taking these medications.

Pharmacokinetics: Metabolized by the liver and excreted through the urine.

Side Effects*:* GI upset, stomatitis, alopecia, uric acid increased, photosensitivity, headache, and hepatotoxicity.

Nursing Care: Monitor labs such as CBC, platelets, WBC, uric acid, electrolytes, LFTs, and renal function. Administer antiemetics before administration. Methotrexate is often administered with leucovorin to prevent toxicity. Provide oral care such as oral oncology solution. Monitor for toxicity. Maintain fluid intake.

IV. Antitumor Medications

Definition: Antitumor medications affect the cell cycle phase of treatment. These medications interact with DNA to treat cancer. There are two categories—anthracyclines, which can cause damage to the heart, and nonanthracyclines, which do not cause damage to the heart.

Types: Anthracyclines are doxorubicin (Adriamycin) and daunorubicin (Cerubidine). Nonanthracyclines are dactinomycin (Actinimycin), bleomycin (Blenoxane), and mitomycin (Mutamycin).

Contraindications: Patients with cardiac conditions should use caution when taking these medications.

Pharmacokinetics: Given IV; metabolized by the liver and excreted through the bile or liver.

Side Effects: GI upset, cardiac dysthymias, heart failure, bone marrow suppression, nausea, vomiting, anemia, stomatitis, hair loss, increased uric acid, and cardiotoxicity.

Nursing Care: Obtain health history before administering. Monitor for cardiotoxicity. Obtain labs such as CBC, platelets, and electrolytes before administration. Administer an antiemetic before administration. Continue to monitor for complications. Increase fluid intake, and maintain a healthy diet. Cardiac monitoring may be needed.

V. Vinca Alkaloids/Taxanes

Definition: **These medications are mitotic inhibitors that prevent miosis, resulting in decreased cell division and cell death.** ←

Types: Vinca alkaloids are vincristine (Oncovin), vinorelbine (Navelbine), and vinblastine (Velban). Taxanes are paclitaxel (Abraxane, Onxol, Taxol) and docetaxel (Taxotere).

Contraindications: Patients with renal or liver disease should use caution when taking these medications.

Pharmacokinetics: Given IV; metabolized by the liver and excreted through the bile.

Side Effects: **GI upset, weight loss, peripheral neuropathy, weakness, neutropenia, alopecia, stomatitis, ptosis, neurotoxicity, hypotension, bronchospasm, rash, and cardiac problems.** ←

Nursing Care: Monitor LFTs. Assess for CNS changes. Administer in a 24-hour infusion. Cardiac monitoring is needed. Monitor vital signs. Assess respiratory status.

VI. Topoisomerase Inhibitors

Definition: These medications prevent DNA synthesis and replication. Cell cycle phase–specific treatment.

Types: Topotecan (Hycamtin), etoposide (VePesid, Toposar, Etopophos), irinotecan (Camptosar), and teniposide (Vumon).

Contraindication: Patients with liver and renal disease should use caution when taking these medications.

Pharmacokinetics: Given PO or IV. Metabolized by the liver and excreted through the urine and bile.

→ *Side Effects:* **Bone marrow suppression, GI upset, alopecia, stomatitis, headache, diarrhea, weight loss, abdominal cramping, hypotension, anemia, rash, and thrombocytopenia.**

Nursing Care: Monitor labs and vital signs before administration. Teach the patient about side effects and complications that can arise when taking this medication. Encourage the patient to increase fluid intake and maintain a healthy diet.

VII. Antiestrogens

Definition: Antiestrogens block estrogen receptors and inhibit tumor growth. They are used to treat breast cancer.

Types: Anastrozole (Arimidex), tamoxifen (Nolvadex), raloxifene (Evista), exemestane (Aromasin), letrozole (Femara), fulvestrant (Faslodex), and toremifene (Fareston).

Contraindications: Patients with liver and renal disease should use caution when taking these medications.

Pharmacokinetics: Given PO or IV. Metabolized by the liver and excreted through the urine or bile.

Side Effects: Hot flashes, vaginal discharge, sweating, GI upset, dizziness, hypercalcemia, headache, bone pain, and fatigue.

Nursing Care: Monitor labs and vital signs. Teach the patient the side effects that can occur with this medication. Encourage fluid intake. A mastectomy may also be performed in conjunction with this medication.

Hematopoietic Growth Factors

Definition: These products are used as supportive therapy in patients with some cancers of the blood.

Types: Erythropoetin (Epogen) and filgrastim (Neupogen).

Contraindications: Patients with cardiac problems should use caution when taking these medications.

Pharmacokinetics: Metabolized by the liver.

Side Effects: Hypertension, fluid retention, bone pain, and cardiac changes.

Nursing Care: **When patients become neutropenic (WBC <10,000) these products are given to increase white blood cell production and increase immune support**. Monitor labs daily. Use neutropenic precautions when caring for these patients. ←

Antibiotics

Definition: These medications are used to prevent or inhibit bacterial growth that can lead to infections, or to treat existing infections.

Types:

- Penicillin: Amoxicillin (Amoxil), ampicillin (Principil), carbenicillin (Geocillin), and oxacillin (Bactocill).
- Aminoglycosides: Streptomycin, gentamicin, tobramycin, and neomycin.
- Sulfonamides: Trimethoprim/sulfamethoxazole.
- Cephalosporin: Cephalexin (Keflex), cefdinir (Omnicef), and ceftriaxone (Rocephin).
- Fluoroquinolone: Ciprofloxacin, levofloxacin, and gemifloxacin.
- Tetracycline: Doxycycline and minocycline.
- Macrolides: Azithromycin, erythromycin, and clarithromycin.

Contraindications: Obtain an allergy history before administering, and do not give if there has been a prior allergic response.

Pharmacokinetics: Given PO or IV; metabolized by the liver and excreted through the urine.

Side Effects: Headache, GI upset, hepatotoxicity, nephrotoxicity, allergic reactions, rash, and drowsiness. With sulfonamides, Stevens–Johnson's syndrome can be a side effect.

Nursing Care: Obtain an allergy history before administering. Monitor for side effects. Administer a probiotic to avoid complications such as *C. diff.* Monitor labs.

PAIN MANAGEMENT

Opioid Analgesics

Definition: These medications control pain by blocking pain receptors in the brain.

Types: Morphine sulfate, fentanyl, meperidine (Demerol), hydromorphone (Dilaudid), oxycodone/acetaminophen (Percocet), oxycodone (Oxycontin), codeine, and tramadol (Ultram).

Contraindications: Obtain an allergy history before administering. Patients with depressed respirations and bradycardia should use caution when taking these medications. Use with caution in patients who are sedated or drowsy.

Pharmacokinetics: Given PO or IV. Metabolized by the liver and excreted through the urine.

Side Effects: Drowsiness, nausea, vomiting, hypotension, urinary retention, constipation, respiratory depression, and impaired vision.

Nursing Care: Teach the patient about the side effects of the → medications. **Monitor the patient's mental status. Narcan can be given if the patient is overmedicated**. Monitor vital signs. Advise patients to avoid alcohol while taking these medications. Opioids can also be given through a patient-controlled analgesic device. To decrease constipation, use stool softeners daily. Encourage patients to take these medications with food to avoid GI upset.

Nonopioid Analgesics

Definition: These medications have anti-inflammatory, antipyretic, and pain-relieving effects.

Types: Acetaminophen (Tylenol) and ibuprofen (Motrin).

Contraindications: Patients with liver disease should not use these medications.

Pharmacokinetics: Given PO; metabolized by the liver and excreted by the kidneys.

Side Effects: GI upset, hearing loss, liver and renal toxicity.

Nursing Care: Advise patients to take medication with food to decrease GI upset. Monitor renal and liver tests before administration. Monitor for tinnitus. Teach the patient the side effects of the medication. Always use a pain scale to assess pain. Recheck the pain level in 15 minutes.

PEDIATRIC NURSING

SIX

Let us take time out and escape the world of adult health and enter the world of pediatrics. Pediatric patients tend to be a little happier, full of life, and excited about everything. Patients vary in age from babies to 17-year-olds. Most inpatient care units are colorful and have activity rooms for little patients to play in. Although the cases are often sad and no one wants to see kids sick, providing care and helping them feel better makes it all worthwhile. Playing games, such as peek-a-boo, dressing up, and putting together puzzles, are just part of what your day might consist of. The best part about our job as nurses is that we can help and play at the same time.

In the pediatric nursing course, you learn about the stages of development, common disorders, treatments, and nursing interventions. This chapter has the same set-up as that of Chapter 3. Each disorder will be explained in detail with highlighted areas to concentrate on. The course exams will be based on learning the various conditions and recognizing the nursing interventions for each. There are many questions on child development stages as well. Medication administration and dosage of medications are also slightly different. Study your medication calculations for pediatric dosing.

I found this course to be a nice change from adult care nursing, but a little bit difficult, due to the abundance of information. Now, you may have a totally different experience—don't begin to worry yet. This course is packed with lots of information and requires lots of studying, as well. The clinical portion of the course will test your knowledge and what you have learned. Assessment, care plans, knowledge of medication dosages, and nursing interventions are all part of your clinical experience. Pediatric patients endure the same severity of symptoms as adult patients. Clinical placements can vary. It may be emotionally difficult for you to see children suffering from illness. But as a nursing student, you have to remember you are there to help these kids feel better. Once a child smiles at you and says a simple "thank you," you will begin to see the beauty in caring for children.

My pediatric clinical experience took place in Boston Children's Hospital on the cystic fibrosis unit. I was amazed. The unit was very colorful and vibrant, and all the rooms looked like mini toy shops. Although the kids were sick and weak, they were full of life and ready to play. The day begins with administering morning medications, completing assessments, and reviewing the chart. Once this was completed, it was time to play! I would often say to myself, "Now, this is a dream nursing job!"

I hope you enjoy this course and clinical as much as I did. Pay attention to the check boxes on the margins; they highlight areas that were frequently tested. The first exam will be based on knowing the different developmental stages; this content is also tested on the NCLEX. The next three to four exams are based on pediatric medications, review of disorders, and nursing interventions. You can apply the same study skills from the prior courses to study for this course. Let's get started!

PEDIATRIC PHYSICAL ASSESSMENT

The assessment of a child is similar to that of the adult. You want to start your assessment from head to toe in order to get a general overall appearance of the patient. When obtaining a health history, the parents are usually the ones who are going to give you all the information. Explain each step to the parents so they are aware and comfortable, as well. Obtain vital signs and use the FLACC scale to assess pain. In the case of patients who are too young to express how they are feeling, asking the parents the symptoms or the child's usual behavior may help. This is the most difficult part of pediatric nursing: although adults can tell you how they feel, often times children cannot. A thorough assessment is vital in order to diagnose and treat the patient. Remember, the parents' consent is needed at all times. Always obtain a health history before beginning the assessment.

Vital Signs

Vital signs are different for infants, children, and adolescents. You will be tested on knowing the difference.

I. Temperature

An accurate axillary, oral, rectal, or tympanic temperature is obtained. An oral temperature should only be obtained from children who are 4 years of age or older. For patients 1 to 3 years old, temperature is taken tympanically. Rectal temperatures are used for newborns and infants up to a year old. The normal temperature for a child is 98.6°F.

II. Pulse

To obtain the heart rate, the apical pulse is palpated and assessed for a full minute. The brachial pulse can be used on older children. It is important to also document the child's activity level at the time of assessment. Was the child crying, screaming, or running around? The normal range of pulse is:

Birth: 100 to 170 bpm

3 to 6 months: 100 to 120 bpm

6 to 12 months: 80 to 120 bpm

1 to 3 years: 70 to 110 bpm

3 to 6 years: 60 to 110 bpm

6 to 12 years: 60 to 90 bpm

12 years to adult: 60 to 100 bpm

III. Blood Pressure

The blood pressure (BP) is taken with a pediatric cuff. The normal range of blood pressure (systolic/diastolic) is:

Birth to 3 months: 60 to 80 mmHg/40 to 50 mmHg

3 to 6 months: 70 to 90 mmHg/50 to 60 mmHg

6 to 12 months: 80 to 100 mmHg/50 to 60 mmHg

1 to 3 years: 90 to 100 mmHg/60 to 70 mmHg

3 to 6 years: 95 to 110 mmHg/60 to 75 mmHg

6 to 12 years: 100 to 120 mmHg/60 to 80 mmHg

12 years to adult: 110 to 130 mmHg/65 to 85 mmHg

IV. Respirations

Infants have diaphragmatic respirations, so it is important to use the abdomen to assess respiratory rates. Count the respirations for a full minute, and document your findings, also assessing for any complications or changes. The normal respiratory rate is:

Birth to 6 months: 30 to 55 breaths per minute.

6 months to 12 months: 35 to 45 breaths per minute

1 to 3 years: 20 to 30 breaths per minute

3 to 6 years: 20 to 25 breaths per minute

6 to 12 years: 14 to 20 breaths per minute

12 years to adult: 12 to 18 breaths per minute

V. Pain

When assessing for pain, assess the infant's behavioral response. Is the child crying or squirming around? Does the infant's response to pain increase with palpation of the affected area? If the child is old enough to tell you where the pain is, assess the area and treat.

Head and Neck

Observe the head for shape and symmetry. Palpate the skull, assessing for any lesions, fractures, or swelling. Palpate the anterior and posterior fontanels. The anterior fontanel closes at 12 to 18 months. In older children, the posterior fontanel is assessed.

Place the child in a sitting position to assess the neck. Assess ROM (moving the neck side to side). Assess for any lesions, skin folds, or swelling. Palpate the trachea. Document any findings.

Eyes and Ear Assessment

Inspect the eyes and lids for symmetry. Inspect the conjunctiva, which should appear pink and glossy. Inspect the sclera, which should appear white and clear. A yellow tint of the sclera can signify jaundice. If the child can follow directions, assess the extraocular movement by evaluating the cardinal fields of gaze.

Inspect the ears for symmetry. Note if there are any abnormalities, pain, or drainage. Observe the tympanic membrane. Palpate the mastoid for tenderness. Assess for signs of an ear infection. To assess hearing acuity for infants, clap to elicit a response. For school-age children, a whisper test is conducted. Document any findings.

Face, Nose, Mouth, and Throat

Observe the face for symmetry. Any deviation can be caused by nerve damage. Observe the nose for symmetry. Flaring of the nares can indicate respiratory failure. Observe the internal nasal cavity for discharge and swelling.

Inspect the lips for swelling and lesions. Assess the tonsils; if reddened, they can signify an infection. Palpate the neck for any lesions or abnormalities. Inspect the oral mucosa, gums, tongue, and teeth. Count the number of teeth, and if the child is at the relevant age, check for loose teeth. Use a tongue blade to assist in the exam. Do not use a tongue blade if the patient is experiencing epiglottitis. Document the findings.

Thorax and Lungs

Inspect the thorax for symmetry. Assess for any abnormalities. A barrel-shaped chest can indicate respiratory problems. Measure the chest, making sure there are no deviations. Assess the thorax for any abnormalities. Labored breathing or cyanosis can indicate respiratory difficulty. Listen for breath sounds. Auscultate the lung fields. Document the findings.

Cardiovascular Assessment

Place the child in a sitting position if possible; infants can remain in the lying position. Inspect for cyanosis of the fingers or feet. Assess for edema, looking for signs of fluid overload. Assess capillary refill and pulses. Auscultate the heart sounds with a stethoscope. Assess for murmurs or irregular heartbeats. Document your findings.

Abdomen

Inspect the abdomen, assessing for pain or any abnormalities. Inspect the umbilicus; an umbilical hernia is common in infants. Auscultate the four quadrants, making sure to hear active bowel sounds. Palpate the abdomen. Assess for tenderness, enlarged spleen or liver, and distended bladder. Document the findings.

Reproductive System and Assessment

Inspect the breast for size, symmetry, and color. Palpate the breast tissue for any lumps or lesions. Inspect the pubis for hair growth. For girls, assess the labia for any redness or swelling. Adolescents may be guarded and want to maintain their privacy. Ask adolescent girls if they have started their menstrual cycle. For boys, assess the penis for any swelling or abnormalities. With adolescents, ask about sexual activity as well. Always obtain consent from the parent, and explain the assessment step by step. Document the findings.

Musculoskeletal Assessment

Inspect the spine, assessing for scoliosis. The spine should appear straight with no deviations. Inspect the upper extremities, bones, and joints. Assess muscle strength by having the child squeeze your hand. Assess the bilateral lower extremities for strength. Ask the child to walk in a straight line. Assess for unsteady gait or difficulty walking. In infants, make sure the legs are aligned. Assess ROM. Document the findings.

Neurological Assessment

Assess level of consciousness. Assess the cranial nerves (refer to Chapter 2). Assess the child's motor function and sensory function. Document the findings.

Growth and Development

This section is very important! The first exam is based on the growth and development of the child. From birth through adolescence, we will review each developmental stage.

Infants

First assess the weight and height of the infant. Infants gain 5 to 7 ounces per week. By 6 months, the weight has doubled. By the first year, the weight has tripled. The height increases 1 inch per month for the first 6 months.

Fine motor development improves rapidly from the age of 2 months to 1 year. Grasping objects begins at 2 to 3 months. Transferring objects from one hand to the other starts at 7 months. At the age of 10 months, the infant is able to use the pincer grasp. Infants begin removing objects from containers at 11 months. They begin to build block towers at the age of 1 year.

Gross motor development begins with head control and progresses to the sitting position. Infants begin to roll over at 4 to 6 months. They are able to sit alone at the age of 7 months. At 10 months, they transition themselves from the prone to the sitting position. At the age of 6 to 7 months, infants begin to crawl. Between 12 and 14 months, infants start to walk. Each child develops differently, and these developmental milestones can vary with each child.

Cognitive development is evaluated based on the theory developed by Jean Piaget. At the end of the first year, infants develop the concept of object permanence. Separation anxiety occurs. By the age of 1, the child begins to learn a few words.

Infants start eating solid foods at 6 months. Introduce food at intervals to assess for allergies. Infants should be placed on their back to sleep. Injury preventions need to be initiated, especially when infants start to crawl and walk.

Toddlers (12 to 36 Months)

Weight gain begins to slow down, averaging a 4- to 6-pound increase a year. The birth weight is quadrupled by the age of 2 years. Height increases by an average of 3 inches per year. The five senses begin to develop. Toddlers are active and explore their environment.

Gross and fine motor skills become more defined and developed. Toddlers are able to build towers and throw a ball at 18 months. They develop skills such as putting on their shoes and are ready for toilet training.

Psychosocial development is evaluated using Erik Erikson's theory regarding the development of autonomy. According to Erikson, maintaining a daily ritual for the toddler provides comfort. Toddlers are able to separate themselves from their parents and begin to interact with other children. Cognitive development is assessed using Piaget's sensorimotor and preconception phases. By age 2, toddlers are able to differentiate sexes and name their body parts.

Toddlers should begin regular dental and medical checkups. We all know this age as the "terrible twos," so safety is important. All medications and cleaning supplies should be kept out of reach.

Preschool (3 to 5 Years)

The average preschooler gains 5 pounds a year. Height increases 2 to 3 inches a year. Gross motor activity includes walking, running, jumping, and climbing. Fine motor activities include drawing and beginning to write. Psychosocial development according to Erikson's theory centers on the child's sense of initiative. Feelings of guilt develop along with the superego. Preschool age children begin to learn right from wrong and recognize the consequences of their actions.

School-Age Children (6 to 12 Years)

During this stage, height increases by 2 inches per year. The body begins to change and mature. Psychological development is evaluated using Piaget's and Erikson's theories. Piaget stated that during this stage school-age children use *conceptual thinking*. Erikson's phase of inferiority also applies to this age group. Children begin to take on more tasks in which they may or may not succeed, which increases feelings of inferiority. School-age children identify with their peers. Team play and social activities are important during this age. Engagement in extracurricular activities begins.

Adolescents (13 to 18 Years)

During this stage, the body begins to develop from a child to an adult. Puberty begins for both boys and girls. Girls begin menstruation. Boys begin to see an increase in hair growth along with voice changes. Height and weight both slightly increase. Psychosocial development is evaluated using Erikson's theory, which focuses on attaining a sense of identity. Adolescents seek to find out who they are. Piaget stated that adolescents begin to use abstract thinking to make decisions.

Work and social activities are important to adolescents. Teach the importance of safety. Motor vehicle accidents are the leading cause of death for this age group. The ramifications of alcohol and drug abuse need to be taught. Safe sexual activity should also be discussed. Adolescents tend to rely less on their parents and take guidance from their peers.

CARDIOVASCULAR DISORDERS

Increased Pulmonary Blood Flow Defects

Definition: In this defect, there is a disruption of blood flow between the vessels and the septum, resulting in a cardiac defect. There is an increased blood flow to the right side of the heart, causing signs of congestive heart failure. Three types of disorders can occur: atrial septal defect, ventricular septal defect, and patent ductus arteriosus.

Atrial Septal Defect

Definition: Infants with atrial septal defect have an open atria and septum that is incomplete.

Signs and Symptoms: Asymptomatic, fluid overload, edema, crackles upon auscultation, shortness of breath, heart murmur, and dysrhythmias.

Treatment: Can close on its own without the need for surgery. If atrial opening does not close, a cardiopulmonary bypass is performed before the age of 6. A cardiac catheterization may also be needed to facilitate closing.

Ventricular Septal Defect

Definition: Caused by an abnormal opening between the right and left ventricles.

Signs and Symptoms: Asymptomatic, heart murmur, signs of congestive heart failure, fatigue, and loss of appetite.

Treatment: Most ventricular septal defects close on their own. Cardiac catheterization can be done. If there is no closure, a cardiopulmonary bypass is performed. Surgery is typically done before age 2.

Patent Ductus Arteriosus

Definition: Opening between the aorta and the pulmonary artery.

Signs and Symptoms: Asymptomatic, heart murmur, signs of CHF, strong bounding pulse, and fatigue.

Treatment: Administration of indomethacin can help with closure. If ineffective, cardiac catheterization is performed. In severe cases, surgery is needed, and a thoracotomy is performed.

Obstructive Cardiac Defects

Definition: In this defect, the blood exits the heart and stenosis occurs, causing an obstruction of blood flow. The obstruction causes a decrease in cardiac output. There are three types of stenosis: coarctation of aorta, pulmonic stenosis, and aortic stenosis.

I. Coarctation of the Aorta

Definition: The opening of the aorta is narrowed and obstructed.

Signs and Symptoms: Increased blood pressure, signs of CHF, bounding pulse, headache, dizziness, and nosebleeds.

Treatment: Balloon angioplasty can help with closure. If this is not effective, surgery is needed to resect the coarcted portion with end-to-end anastomosis of the aorta. Hypertensive medications may be needed to treat the increase in blood pressure.

II. Pulmonic Stenosis

Definition: This is a narrowing of the pulmonary artery, which can cause right ventricular hypertrophy.

Signs and Symptoms: Asymptomatic, cardiac murmur, cyanosis, and severe CHF.

Treatment: Balloon angioplasty through cardiac catheterization to open the obstructed artery. If this is ineffective, a transventricular valvotomy procedure is performed.

III. Aortic Stenosis

Definition: This is a narrowing of the aortic valve that results in left ventricular hypertrophy.

Signs and Symptoms: Pulmonary edema, increased heart rate, hypotension, decreased cardiac output, dizziness, cardiac murmur, CHF, and cyanosis.

Treatment: Balloon angioplasty through cardiac catheterization; if this is ineffective, surgery is needed.

Decreased Pulmonary Blood Flow Defects

Definition: In these defects, pulmonary blood flow is obstructed between the right and the left ventricles. Tetralogy of Fallot is a common condition.

Tetralogy of Fallot

Definition: This comprises a combination of four defects, namely, ventricular septal defect, pulmonic stenosis, overriding aorta, and right ventricular hypertrophy.

→ *Signs and Symptoms:* **Cyanosis, hypoxemia, heart murmur, clubbing, "tet spells" (cyanosis occurs when bathing or feeding). A common symptom is the occurrence of a "tet spell," in which the child is in a tripod position.**

Treatment: A shunt can be placed to increase blood flow. If this is ineffective, a complete repair is needed. This involves a medial sternotomy and the use of cardiopulmonary bypass. Treatment for "tet spells" is morphine, oxygen, and fluids.

Mixed Cardiac Defects

Definition: Cardiac defects occur where mixing of the blood takes place. Saturated blood flow mixes with unsaturated blood flow, causing pulmonary congestion and decreased cardiac output. The three types of mixed cardiac defects are transposition of the great arteries, hypoplastic left heart syndrome, and total anomalous pulmonary venous connection.

I. Transposition of Great Arteries

Definition: The pulmonary artery leaves the left ventricle and the aorta, which expels the blood from the right ventricle.

Signs and Symptoms: Cyanosis, CHF, and cardiomegaly.

Treatment: Prostaglandin E can be given to keep the patent ductus arteriosus open. A balloon atrial septostomy is performed to increase cardiac output. Surgical treatment consists of an arterial switch whereby normal circulation is increased.

II. Hypoplastic Left Heart Syndrome

→ *Definition:* This occurs when **the left side of the heart is not fully developed and causes both hypoplastic left heart syndrome and aortic atresia.**

Signs and Symptoms: Cyanosis, CHF, shock, and hypotension. The condition needs to be treated immediately, or death can occur.

Treatment: A heart transplant is needed. Before surgery, the infant is treated with prostaglandin E, and mechanical ventilation is used until the transplant is done.

III. Total Anomalous Pulmonary Venous Connection

Definition: Blood flow is obstructed between the pulmonary veins and the left atrium.

Signs and Symptoms: Cyanosis, small heart size, CHF, and pulmonary congestion.

Treatment: Surgery is needed, and the atrial septal defect is closed, and the pulmonary veins are reconnected to the left atrium.

Congestive Heart Failure (CHF)

Definition: CHF is the inability of the heart to provide enough blood and oxygen to the body. The common cause of CHF in children is congenital heart defects. The child can suffer from either right- or left-sided heart failure.

Signs and Symptoms: **Left-sided heart failure symptoms are wheezing, crackles, dyspnea, respiratory distress, nasal flaring, retractions, increased respirations, and cough. Right-sided heart failure symptoms are peripheral edema, weight gain, fluid overload, ascites, hepatomegaly, and jugular vein distension.** ←

Diagnostics: Presentation of symptoms, chest x-ray, and labs.

Complications: If left untreated, respiratory distress and severe hypoxemia can occur. Digoxin toxicity can also occur if a toxic level is reached.

Drug Therapy: Oxygen administration, diuretics, digoxin, potassium infusion, and angiotensin-converting enzyme inhibitors are given.

Nursing Care: Maintain a patent airway. Monitor vital signs, labs, strict intake/output, daily weights, and fluid intake. Keep the HOB elevated, and administer oxygen if needed. Monitor digoxin levels and monitor for toxicity. Diuretics are administered, and electrolytes are monitored during this treatment. Keep the child in a quiet, calm environment. **Comfort the child; crying and excessive activity can cause the child to become cyanotic and short of breath.** ← With right-sided heart failure, fluid restriction and constant monitoring of fluid intake is needed.

Endocarditis

→ *Definition:* **Infection of the valves and the lining of the heart. It is caused by *Staphylococcus* and *Streptococcus* agents.** Children with congenital heart defects or rheumatic heart disease are at risk for endocarditis.

→ *Signs and Symptoms:* **Fever, weight loss, Osler lesions, Janeway lesions, weakness, and fatigue.**

Diagnostics: Increased WBC levels, positive blood cultures, and echocardiographic abnormalities.

Drug Therapy: IV antibiotics are given to treat endocarditis. To prevent endocarditis in children who are at risk, always administer an antibiotic before any dental or surgical procedures.

Nursing Care: Monitor labs and vital signs. Assess for fever every 4 hours and treat as ordered. Teach the patient preventive measures such as taking antibiotics before procedures. Long-term antibiotics may be needed. The child needs to be closely monitored by the physician, with frequent checkups.

Rheumatic Fever

Definition: This is an inflammatory autoimmune disease that affects the heart, joints, skin, and brain. It is secondary to strep. Rheumatic fever commonly occurs 2 to 6 weeks after the initial infection. The Jones criteria are used to diagnose the progression of the disease.

Signs and Symptoms: Major symptoms include carditis, polyarthritis, erythema marginatum, chorea, and subcutaneous nodules. Carditis includes increased heart rate, chest pain, pericardial friction, murmurs, and inflammation of the valves. Erythema marginatum is characterized by red lesions on the abdomen and extremities. Chorea is the involuntary movement of the facial and extremity muscles. Speech is also affected. Subcutaneous nodules occur at the joints. Other symptoms are fever, painful joints, cardiac changes, and increased erythrocyte sedimentation rate (ESR).

→ *Diagnostics:* **Jones criteria of symptoms, elevated antistreptolysin O (ASO) titer, elevated ESR, and elevated C-reactive protein (CRP) level.**

Complications: CHF, respiratory failure, and seizures.

Drug Therapy: Antibiotics such as penicillin, antipyretics, and anti-inflammatory medications are given.

Nursing Care: Monitor vital signs and labs. Administer medications as ordered. Treat painful joints with alternation of cold and hot therapy. **Maintain bed rest to conserve energy. Monitor for complications such as seizures and maintain precautions.** If the child is experiencing chorea, maintain safety because of the risk of falls. Teach parents the importance of antibiotic treatment and maintaining a medication schedule.

Kawasaki Disease

Definition: This systemic inflammatory disease commonly occurs in children younger than 5 years old. The cause is unknown.

Signs and Symptoms: **Symptoms depend on the phase of the disease. In the acute phase, symptoms present as swollen hands, irritability, rashes on the trunk, and fever. In the subacute phase, symptoms present as cracking of the lips, joint pain, thrombocytosis, desquamation of the fingers or toes, and a fever that ends after 25 days.**

Diagnostics: Due to the unknown cause, diagnostic testing is used to diagnose this condition. An echocardiogram and lab work are commonly performed.

Complications: Myocardial infarction, shock, and coronary artery aneurysms.

Drug Therapy: **High doses of IV immunoglobulin and aspirin are given.**

Nursing Care: Monitor vital signs and cardiac status. Assess heart sounds, joints, and extremities for swelling. Monitor intake/output and daily weights. Maintain rest to conserve energy. Meals should include soft foods. Administer medications as ordered. Monitor for complications such as CHF, MI, and aneurysms. Teach parents the signs of symptoms and treatment. All immunizations should be deferred for 3 months after symptoms have resolved.

RESPIRATORY DISORDERS

Acute Laryngotracheobronchitis (LTB)

Definition: This is inflammation of the trachea and larynx, which results in edema and narrowing of the airway. Due to the restriction of airflow, respiratory stridor and retractions occur. LTB is commonly known as *croup* and can be either bacterial or viral.

Signs and Symptoms: **Barking cough, stridor, respiratory retractions, distress, fever, cyanosis, increased respirations, and sweating.**

Diagnostics: Based on symptoms. Pulse oximetry and ABGs are obtained.

Complications: Severe airway obstruction and cyanosis.

→ *Drug Therapy:* **A child with mild croup can be treated at home with cool mist with a vaporizer.** If this is not available, steam the bathroom and have the child breathe in mist for a few minutes. Tylenol is given to reduce the fever. Hospitalized children are given corticosteroids, bronchodilators, cough suppressants, nebulizers, and antibiotics.

Nursing Care: Instruct the patient to use cool mist for mild symptoms of croup. If symptoms become severe, hospitalization is required. Rest, increased fluid intake, and respiratory monitoring are done. Have intubation equipment at the bedside. Respiratory difficulty with drooling is a medical emergency and can signify the closing of the airway. Administer medications as ordered by the physician. Instruct the child to conserve energy, with frequent rest periods. Intravenous fluids and oxygen are given. Maintain a patent airway. Decrease anxiety and provide emotional support for both the family and child.

Epiglottitis

Definition: Severe inflammation of the epiglottis, causing → airway obstruction. **This disorder is bacterial and caused by *Haemophilus influenzae*.** It commonly occurs in children 2 to 5 years old and is more prevalent in the winter. This is a life-threatening condition, and immediate care is needed.

→ *Signs and Symptoms:* **Remember the four Ds: drooling, dyspnea, dysphagia, and decreased level of consciousness are common.** Other symptoms include fever, tripod posture, retractions, cyanosis, restlessness, muffled voice, cherry-red throat, tachypnea, increased heart rate, and hypoxia.

Diagnostics: Lateral neck x-ray. A laryngoscopy is done to assess the throat. Remember in cases of epiglottitis, never attempt throat cultures or insertion of airway devices. These assessments and procedures are done only by the physician. Pulse oximetry and ABGs are done.

Complications: Respiratory failure and death.

Drug Therapy: Antibiotics, humidification, corticosteroids, and antipyretics.

→ *Nursing Care:* **If epiglottitis is suspected, intubation or tracheostomy may be performed to maintain an open airway.** Inform the parents that this is temporary. Monitor respiratory status and vital signs closely. Intravenous fluids are administered. Once the respiratory status has improved, the child will be extubated, with close monitoring of respiratory status.

Bronchiolitis or Respiratory Syncytial Virus

Definition: Bronchiolitis is viral infection caused by the respiratory syncytial virus organisms. Inflammation of the bronchi and bronchioles is seen with an increase in mucus production. Airway obstruction is caused by the increased inflammation. It commonly occurs in children younger than 2 years old.

Signs and Symptoms: Cough, wheezing, and rhinorrhea are the first signs. Other symptoms are fever, dyspnea, and apnea. **Severe symptoms are tachypnea, cyanosis, retractions, tachycardia, nasal flaring, grunting, and decreased breath sounds.** ←

Diagnostics: Chest x-ray, WBC, and ELISA test.

Complications: Respiratory failure and death.

Drug Therapy: Ribavirin (Virazole), an antiviral, is used with bronchodilators to treat RSV. Oxygen is also administered.

Nursing Care: Maintain a patent airway and check the level of consciousness. Nebulizers and fluids are administered. **Provide periods of rest to conserve energy.** ← Keep the HOB at a 45° to 90° level to maintain an open airway. Children at risk can be given RSV immunoglobulin.

Pneumonia

Definition: Pneumonia can be viral or bacterial. Inflammation of the pulmonary parenchyma and alveoli occurs. Viral pneumonia is the most common and can be treated at home. Bacterial pneumonia is more severe and requires hospitalization.

Signs and Symptoms: **Cough, crackles, fever, wheezes, cyanosis, irritability, headache, fatigue, shortness of breath, and decreased breath sounds.** ←

Diagnostics: WBC and chest x-ray are performed.

Complications: Pleural effusions and worsening of symptoms.

Drug Therapy: Antipyretics, antibiotics, and cough medication are given.

Nursing Care: Administer oxygen as needed. Administer antibiotics as ordered. Treat fever with antipyretics. Closely monitor vital signs and respiratory status. A humidifier may help facilitate breathing. Monitor for secretions; suctioning may be needed.

Cystic Fibrosis

Definition: This is an autosomal recessive trait disorder. In cystic fibrosis the exocrine gland produces an excessive amount of mucus and secretions. Increased secretions cause respiratory obstruction. Overproduction of the exocrine gland can cause severe electrolyte imbalances.

→ *Signs and Symptoms:* **The earliest sign of CF is meconium ileus, which occurs in newborns. CF affects the respiratory and GI systems. Respiratory symptoms are wheezing, cyanosis, cough, dyspnea, clubbing of the fingers, hypoxemia, barrel chest, and episodes of bronchitis. GI symptoms are abdominal distension, foul-smelling stool, slow growth, weight loss, anemia, dehydration, and deficiency of vitamins A, D, E, and K.**

→ *Diagnostics:* **Sweat chloride tests,** chest x-ray, stool samples, and pulmonary function tests.

Complications: Failure to thrive, respiratory failure, and death.

Drug Therapy: Antibiotics are given through an IV. Pulmozyme, a medication to decrease mucus production, is given. Pancreatic enzymes are given three times a day with meals.

Nursing Care: Chest physiotherapy and nebulizers are administered during the hospital stay and at home to facilitate the expulsion of mucus. Oxygen is administered if needed. Assess lung sounds and report any changes. Administer IVF. Obtain and monitor labs. Maintain a high-calorie diet.

Asthma

Definition: This is a chronic inflammatory condition that causes vasoconstriction of the airways. It can be caused by irritants, smoke, and allergies.

Signs and Symptoms: Wheezing, chest tightness, cough, dyspnea, shortness of breath, restlessness, hypoxemia, barrel chest, and cyanosis. The child may sit in the tripod position to facilitate breathing.

Diagnostics: Presentation of symptoms, pulmonary function tests, and skin testing for allergies.

Complications: **In status asthmaticus the child presents with severe respiratory distress that may result in death. This is a medical emergency.**

Drug Therapy: Corticosteroids, anticholinergics, NSAIDs, beta-adrenergic agonists, leukotriene modifiers, and long-acting bronchodilators are used.

Nursing Care: Maintain a patent airway. Administer medications and oxygen as ordered. Obtain vital signs and labs. Teach both the parent and child how to administer nebulizers at home. Maintain fluids, and during asthma attacks, the child should decrease his or her activity level. Educate the parents and child about the complications.

NEUROLOGICAL DISORDERS

Hydrocephalus

Definition: This is an increase of cerebrospinal fluid (CSF) in the skull. Hydrocephalus can be caused by trauma, hemorrhage, infection, and tumors.

Signs and Symptoms: **Infants present with increased intracranial pressure, anterior fontanel bulging, frontal bossing, restlessness, high-pitched cry, Macewen's sign, and increased head circumference. In children, headache, vomiting, nausea, blurred vision, and seizures can occur. Progressive symptoms of hydrocephalus are a decrease in level of consciousness, Cheyne-Stokes respirations, decerebrate or decorticate positioning, and bradycardia.**

Diagnostics: Neurological examination, Glasgow Coma Scale, and head circumference measurements.

Complications: Seizures and coma.

Drug Therapy: Diuretics, pain management, antiemetics, anticonvulsants, and antibiotics are given.

Nursing Care: Monitor level of consciousness and maintain open airway. Administer medications as ordered. **Surgery is required for placement of a ventriculoperitoneal shunt that drains the fluid from the brain into the peritoneal cavity**. Postoperatively monitor vital signs and neurological status. Maintain HOB at 45°. Position the child on the inoperable side. Monitor intake/output, vital signs, and head circumference. Assess the shunt and monitor for infections. Children are at risk for seizures, and precautions are initiated.

Head Injury

Definition: Open head injury occurs when there is a direct impact or open wound on the skull. Closed head injury is an impaction on the brain, but there is no open wound.

Sign and Symptoms: Early signs of headache, nausea, vomiting, changed level of consciousness, bulging fontanel, high-pitched cry, dizziness, and visual disturbances. **Late signs are decorticate positioning (adduction of arms and legs) and decerebrate (rigid extension of legs/arms).**

Diagnostics: CT/MRI of the brain can show damage to the brain. A lumbar puncture can also be performed.

Complications: Seizures, coma, and death if left untreated.

Drug Therapy: **Osmotic diuretics (Mannitol) to reduce edema, anticonvulsants for seizures, steroids (Decadron) for edema, and pain medication.**

Nursing Care: Monitor vital signs, neurological status, intake, and output. Maintain a patent airway by keeping the head midline and limit activity. Administer medications and IV fluids. Assess the dressing for any drainage. If drainage is present, it needs to be tested for glucose to assess for increased cerebral spinal fluid. Seizure precautions are maintained. If surgery is necessary, preoperative and postoperative education should be given.

Cerebral Palsy

Definition: This is a nonprogressive disorder that consists of impairment of movement and motor skills caused by cerebral injury. The child may also have epilepsy, mental retardation, and hearing or visual loss.

Signs and Symptoms: Poor head control, irritability, feeding difficulty, consistent choking, stiff extremities, involuntary movements, contractures, scissor gait, tremors, and visual changes.

Diagnostics: Cerebral palsy is diagnosed based on the presentation of symptoms.

Complications: Seizures and respiratory aspiration.

Drug Therapy: Baclofen is often given to decrease muscle spasms. Botox is commonly injected into the muscles to increase mobility. Muscle spasms can be painful, and pain medication is given as needed. Anticonvulsants are administered to prevent seizures.

Nursing Care: Maintain seizure, aspiration, and fall precautions. Help the child to achieve his or her maximum potential by providing realistic goals and limits. Arrange for physical, speech, and occupational therapy. To increase mobility, a brace or mobility device may be needed. To prevent aspiration, sit the child upright and hyperextend the neck. A soft food diet may be recommended. Orthopedic surgery may be recommended if the child has a physical deformity, but this is not always the case. Family support and teaching are important because of lifestyle modifications.

Spina Bifida

Definition: This is incomplete closure of the vertebrae caused by a neural tube defect. **There are two types of spina bifida: spina bifida occulta and spina bifida cystica. Spina bifida can be caused by folic acid deficiency, malnutrition, and medications.** ←

Signs and Symptoms: **Clinical manifestations of spina bifida occulta are an abnormal opening of the spine, but the spine does not protrude through the skin. There is a small dimple on the lumbar area. Spina bifida cystica consists of two types—meningocele and myelomeningocele. Meningocele is the protrusion of the meninges due to the incomplete closure; it presents like a sac-like cyst on the lumbar area. Myelomeningocele is the protrusion of meninges, nerves, CSF, and a portion of the spinal cord, which is contained in a sac on the lumbar portion of the back. This form is most severe because of the risk of rupturing the sac, which can lead to complications such as hydrocephalus and infection.** ←

Diagnostics: MRI, CT scan, and myelography can be used to view the brain and spine. Prenatal diagnostics such as alpha-fetoprotein level can be performed. The physician may order a CBC and urine culture.

Complications: Hydrocephalus, paralysis, hemorrhage, infection, joint deformities, and cyanosis.

Drug Therapy: Antibiotics are given preoperatively and postoperatively; pain management postoperatively.

Nursing Care: Monitor vital signs, head circumference, urine output, and neurological status frequently. Surgery is usually performed a few days after birth. If a sac is present, use aseptic techniques to prevent infection, and protect the area with a sterile dressing. The dressing should be changed frequently, diapers are not used, and the child is positioned on his or her abdomen. Prepare the infant for surgery, providing preoperative and postoperative instructions to parents. Most children born with spina bifida have a latex allergy; this needs to be determined before surgery.

Bacterial Meningitis

Definition: Bacterial meningitis is an infection of the central nervous system. Inflammation of the meninges puts the child at a greater risk for hydrocephalus. **This disorder can be caused by various bacterial agents such as *Streptococcus pneumoniae, Neisseria meningitis,* and *E. coli.*** It commonly occurs in school-age children.

Signs and Symptoms: Nuchal rigidity, positive Kernig sign (inability to straighten legs when the hip is flexed), positive Brudzinski sign (neck flexion causes lower extremities to flex), and fever, headache, high-pitched cry, fatigue, photophobia, vomiting, and change in mental status are seen.

Diagnostics: Lumbar puncture for CSF, blood cultures, WBC, and a nasal culture.

Complications: Seizures, hearing loss, mental retardation, brain damage, and nerve dysfunction.

Drug Therapy: High doses of antibiotics, antipyretics, anticonvulsants, antidiuretics, and immunizations.

Nursing Care: The child is placed in an isolation room and is given high doses of antibiotics with IV fluid therapy. Monitor vital signs, intake, output, and neurological status every 2 hours. Decrease stimuli due to photophobia, keeping the room dim and quiet. Monitor for complications.

Reye's Syndrome

Definition: Reye's syndrome is characterized by toxic encephalopathy with fatty deposits in the liver and cerebral edema. It often occurs 7 days after a viral disease. The cause is unknown, but does have a correlation with the use of aspirin and NSAIDs.

Signs and Symptoms: Nausea, vomiting, fatigue, confusion, loss of reflexes, and seizures.

Diagnostics: **LFTs, lumbar puncture, and electroencephalogram.**

Complications: Respiratory arrest and seizures can occur if left untreated.

Drug Therapy: Diuretics, antiemetic, antibiotics, and intravenous fluids.

Nursing Care: Advise parents to use Tylenol as the first line of treatment for children. Avoid aspirin and NSAIDs in young children. Monitor vital signs, neurological status, intake, output, and head circumference. **Keep the room dim and calm, avoiding high levels of stimulation.** Monitor for complications such as increased intracranial pressure and bleeding. Mechanical ventilation may be needed if the child is at risk for respiratory distress.

Seizures

Definition: An imbalance of electrical activity in the brain. There are two types of seizures, generalized and partial. *Generalized seizures* are classified as tonic–clonic (grand mal), in which the child loses consciousness, or absence (petit mal), in which the child briefly loses consciousness. *Partial seizures* are classified as simple, in which there is no loss of consciousness, or complex, in which there is a loss of consciousness.

Signs and Symptoms: With generalized seizures, there is a loss of consciousness, which can be caused by hypoglycemia, stress, or hyperventilation. In a tonic–clonic seizure, the child stiffens and the eyes roll to the back of the head, and violent jerking can occur for several seconds. With partial seizures an aura can occur before the seizure. Absence seizures can display no symptoms, but the child may present with a blank stare or daydreaming.

Diagnostics: Electroencephalogram monitoring of activity in the brain, CT scan, MRI, and CBC are done.

Complications: **Status epilepticus is a seizure that lasts longer than 30 minutes and can cause severe brain damage. This is a medical emergency and is treated with IV valium.**

Drug Therapy: Anticonvulsants such as carbamazepine (Tegretol), phenytoin (Dilantin), and gabapentin (Neurontin) are used to control seizures.

Nursing Care: Maintain safety and initiate seizure precautions. Maintain a patent airway and keep intubation kit at the bedside. If the child has a seizure, maintain a patent airway, ensure safety by loosening any restrictive clothing, and remove any equipment surrounding the child. Pad the side rails as well. Time the seizure and document the episode. A ketogenic diet may be initiated by decreasing levels of carbohydrates and fat that can cause seizures. Administer medications as ordered. Educate the family about seizure precautions and treatments.

ENDOCRINE DISORDERS

Hypopituitarism (Growth Hormone Deficiency)

Definition: This is caused by a decrease in the secretion of growth hormone (GH) from the pituitary gland. It is commonly caused by autoimmune disorders, tumors, and hereditary or development defects.

Signs and Symptoms: Infants have symptoms of hypoglycemia, increased bilirubin, and delayed skeletal structure. Children have symptoms of slow nail growth, abnormal growth, and high-pitched voice.

Diagnostics: Bone x-rays, assessment of growth patterns, and GH stimulation test.

Drug Therapy: Recombinant human GH is given to replace the hormone.

Nursing Care: Assess growth patterns and treat each complication individually. Family education is needed regarding treatment and home care. Realistic goals need to be set for the child. Teach parents how to administer the recombinant human GH subcutaneously. This injection is given 6 to 7 days a week, and GH levels are frequently monitored.

Hyperpituitarism (Growth Hormone)

Definition: An excessive amount of GH is produced, causing overgrowth of the long bones. This could be caused by a tumor on the pituitary.

→ *Signs and Symptoms:* **Increase in height, overgrowth of facial structures, headache, and increased intracranial pressure.**

Diagnostics: CT scan can show tumor of the pituitary if one is present.

Drug Therapy: Hormone replacement is needed after surgery.

Nursing Care: If a tumor is present, surgery is needed. → **Cryosurgery or hypophysectomy may be performed to remove the tumor**. Preoperative and postoperative teaching is needed. Emotional support is needed as well. Administer hormone replacement medications after surgery.

Precocious Puberty

Definition: Precocious puberty is the development of sexual characteristics before the age of 9 years. It can be caused by disorders of the adrenal glands.

Signs and Symptoms: Breast development, increase in hair growth, acne, headache, and visual disturbances.

Diagnostics: If a tumor is present on the adrenal gland, it can be seen on a CT scan or MRI.

Drug Therapy: **Luteinizing hormone-releasing hormone (Lupron) works by decreasing hormone secretion by the pituitary gland.** ←

Nursing Care: The child may begin to see changes in body image. Teach the patient the proper medication administration and its side effects.

Congenital Hypothyroidism

Definition: This is thyroid deficiency that occurs at birth. It can be caused by defective embryonic development of the thyroid gland or goiter.

Signs and Symptoms: **Jaundice, decreased reflexes, hypothermia, hypotension, anemia, constipation, difficulty feeding, dry skin, coarse hair, abdominal distension, facial edema, depressed nasal bridge, and a large tongue.** ←

Diagnostics: Early detection is important! Monitor levels of thyroid stimulating hormones T3 and T4.

Complications: If not treated early, congenital hypothyroidism can lead to severe mental retardation.

Drug Therapy: Oral thyroid hormone replacements, such as Synthyroid and Levothyroid, can be administered. Pills can be crushed and given through a bottle if needed.

Nursing Care: Lifelong thyroid replacement medications are needed. Parent teaching and home care instructions for medication administration is needed. Early detection is important to decrease the risks of further damage. Continue to monitor for signs of hyperthyroidism. Monitor thyroid hormones frequently while the child is taking this medication.

Diabetes Mellitus

Definition: Type 1 diabetes is caused by a decrease in insulin due to the destruction of pancreatic beta cells. Type 2 diabetes is caused by insulin resistance, which causes insulin deficiency.

Signs of Symptoms: **The "3Ps"—polyuria, polydipsia, and polyphagia**. Other symptoms are fruity breath, headache, weight loss, fatigue, abdominal pain, yeast infections, and fungal infections. ←

Diagnostics: Eight-hour fasting glucose (which can be done at the child's bedtime), urine sample, and blood glucose level.

→ *Complications:* **Diabetic ketoacidosis can occur. Signs and symptoms are fruity breath, Kussmaul respiration, and decreased level of consciousness. This is a medical emergency, and treatment is needed immediately. Other symptoms may include cardiovascular changes, hyperkalemia, and hyperglycemia.**

Drug Therapy: Insulin is needed for treatment. Pediatric dosage of insulin is needed. Types of insulin are short-acting, rapid-acting, intermediate, and long-acting.

Nursing Care: Lifestyle modifications involving diet and exercise are needed. Provide healthy meals with sugar-free snacks. For active children, increase carbohydrates before activities. Blood glucose monitoring is needed. Insulin is administered based on a sliding scale. Assess for signs of hypoglycemia. A school nurse will administer the lunch dose. To treat hypoglycemia, children may carry orange juice or snacks to school. For infants, a blood glucose test is obtained from the heel.

GASTROINTESTINAL DISORDERS

Dehydration

Definition: Imbalance of electrolytes due to the loss of fluid. Dehydration can be caused by diarrhea, vomiting, and infection. Isotonic dehydration is the most common type.

Signs and Symptoms: Sweating, nausea, vomiting, diarrhea, abdominal pain, fever, loss of appetite, metabolic acidosis, and metabolic alkalosis.

Diagnostics: Electrolyte labs.

Complications: Hypovolemic shock can occur with severe dehydration.

Drug Therapy: Oral hydration is first-line treatment. Intravenous fluids may also be administered.

Nursing Care: Monitor labs. Assess the child's vital signs and neurological status. If diarrhea or vomiting is present, assess color and amount. Assess abdomen for distension or pain. Administer intravenous fluids as ordered. Further testing may be needed to treat symptoms. Encourage parents to increase oral hydration if the child is able to tolerate it.

Esophageal Atresia and Tracheoesophageal Fistula

Definition: Esophageal atresia and tracheoesophageal fistula (TEF) are congenital defects that result in a separation between the trachea and the esophagus. This occurs between 6 and 8 weeks of gestation. Due to this separation, all feedings enter the lungs and cause respiratory aspiration.

Signs and Symptoms: **The three Cs—coughing, choking, and cyanosis**. Cyanosis occurs with feedings. Other symptoms include abdominal distension, increased saliva, vomiting, and apnea.

Diagnostics: Clinical symptoms and x-rays of the abdomen are done.

Complications: Aspiration pneumonia, respiratory distress, and death.

Drug Therapy: Antibiotics, antiemetic, and pain management.

Nursing Care:

Surgery is needed if esophageal atresia or tracheoesophageal fistula is suspected. Preoperatively, the child remains NPO with continuous suction of secretions. Keep the HOB at a 45° to 90° angle. Administer intravenous fluids. Assess for aspiration and fevers. The surgical procedure is a thoracotomy with an end-to-end anastomosis of the esophagus. A gastrostomy may also be performed if the infant is premature.

Postoperatively, care consists of assessing the child's respiratory status and vital signs. Suction remains on low continuous. Administer intravenous fluids, antibiotics, and parenteral nutrition. A chest tube may be present; assess drainage. Monitor labs and signs of infection. As the child recovers, solid food and oral intake is implemented slowly. Family education and support is provided.

Pyloric Stenosis

Definition: Pyloric stenosis occurs when the muscles surrounding the pyloric sphincter thicken, resulting in gastric emptying obstruction. Narrowing of the pyloric canal between the stomach and the duodenum occurs.

Signs and Symptoms: **Projectile vomiting, olive-shaped mass in the right upper abdominal quadrant, dehydration, weight loss, vomiting after feeding, electrolyte imbalance, and metabolic alkalosis.**

Diagnostics: **Olive-shaped mass** is seen on x-ray and lab work is obtained.

Drug Therapy: Antibiotics, antiemetics, and IV fluids are administered.

Nursing Care: A pyloromyotomy is performed to treat pyloric stenosis. IV fluids, labs, antibiotics, and vital signs are closely monitored preoperatively. If an NGT is needed, continuous suctioning may be needed to remove excess gastric secretions. Educate parents about what to expect before and after surgery. Continue to monitor the child closely for any complications.

Intussusception

Definition: An acute bowel obstruction at the ileocecal junction. Ischemia of the bowel tissue occurs.

→ *Signs and Symptoms:* **Currant jelly stools, abdominal pain, sausage-shaped mass in the upper right quadrant, vomiting, and decreased bowel sounds.**

Diagnostics: A barium enema and ultrasound of the bowels. CBC, electrolytes, and NGT for decompression of the bowel are also used.

Complications: Ischemia of the bowel can occur if left untreated.

Drug Therapy: Antibiotics, pain management, and intravenous fluids.

Nursing Care: Monitor the child for complications. Administer IV fluids and antibiotics as ordered. NGT is low continuous suction; monitor output every shift. Monitor labs and vital signs. Once stool is brown and formed, a diet is slowly introduced.

Hirschsprung's Disease

Definition: A congenital aganglionic colon disorder in which a distal bowel obstruction occurs. Due to the decrease in ganglionic cells, there is no peristalsis.

→ *Signs and Symptoms:* **Meconium stool is delayed during the first 24 hours.** Other symptoms include abdominal distension, ribbon-like stool, loss of appetite, decreased bowel sounds, diarrhea, weight loss, and failure to thrive.

Diagnostics: A barium enema is given and a rectal biopsy obtained.

Complications: Ischemia of the bowel, which can lead to enterocolitis.

Drug Therapy: Stool softeners and enemas are given for treatment.

Nursing Care: A bowel resection may be performed to resolve the obstruction. A temporary colostomy may be placed until bowel function returns. Administer IV fluids and antibiotics as ordered. Daily weights and abdominal girth are assessed. Postoperatively monitor vital signs and signs of infection. The child remains NPO with an NGT. Parenteral nutrition is administered. A stoma will be created for stool excretion, and a colostomy is bag is placed over the stoma. Teach the parents colostomy care.

Gastrointestinal Reflux

Definition: Gastrointestinal reflux occurs when gastric contents enter the esophagus due to an immature esophageal sphincter.

Signs and Symptoms: Vomiting, irritability, heartburn, anemia, abdominal pain, and regurgitation.

Diagnostics: Barium swallow is given, and a CT of the abdomen may be needed.

Complications: Esophagitis and aspiration pneumonia can occur.

Drug Therapy: **H2 antagonists (Pepcid or Tagamet) and proton pump inhibitors decrease acid production.**

Nursing Care: Infants spit up formula feedings frequently when GERD occurs. To prevent regurgitation, hold infants head up after feedings. Monitor intake and output. Administer medications as ordered. If symptoms worsen or are not resolved, surgery may be needed. A fundoplication or gastrostomy is performed.

Appendicitis

Definition: Inflammation of the appendix.

Signs and Symptoms: Abdominal pain, fever, nausea, rebound tenderness, pain in the right lower quadrant, and **positive McBurney's sign.**

Diagnostics: CT of the abdomen, CBC, WBC, and ultrasound of the abdomen.

Complications: Ruptured appendix and sepsis.

Drug Therapy: Antibiotics, antipyretics, and pain management.

Nursing Care: A surgical appendectomy is performed. Preoperative and postoperative teaching is needed. Monitor vital signs, labs, and pain. Administer medications as ordered. Place the child in semi-Fowler's position to decrease discomfort. **Never administer laxatives or apply heat to the abdomen.**

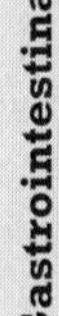

Postoperatively monitor the site and control pain. Administer antibiotics. A drain may be placed to remove excess fluids. Monitor for complications.

Omphalocele and Gastroschisis

Definition: *Gastroschisis* is a defect in the thickness of the abdominal wall near the umbilicus, exposing the abdominal contents. *Omphalocele* is protrusion of the intestines through the abdominal wall. A protruding sac of organs is visible, covered with a clear membrane.

Signs and Symptoms: An abdominal wall defect (gastroschisis) or protruding sac (omphalocele) is usually identified at birth. These defects cause discomfort, and the infant is at risk for infection and damage to the internal organs.

Diagnostics: Based on the presence of symptoms.

Drug Therapy: Antibiotics and pain management.

Nursing Care: In gastroschisis, the abdominal wall defect is covered with saline-soaked gauze, and surgery is immediately performed. For patients with omphalocele, the intestines are covered to protect against infection. Nurses must do dressing changes every shift and protect the site until surgery is completed. Prevention of infection is key. Administer antibiotics as ordered. Provide parents with postoperative and preoperative teaching.

Imperforate Anus

Definition: This results from incomplete development of the anus during gestation.

Signs and Symptoms: Abdominal distension and stool impaction.

Diagnostics: Abdominal ultrasound and CT of the abdomen.

Complications: A bowel obstruction can occur if left untreated.

Drug Therapy: Antibiotics and IVF administration.

Nursing Care: A bowel resection is surgically needed. Preoperative and postoperative nursing management is needed. Maintain hydration. A colostomy may be placed temporarily. Avoid rectal temperatures. Continue to monitor for complications.

Cleft Lip and Palate

Definition: Cleft lip and palate are congenital facial abnormalities that occur when the tissues of the lip and nose fail to develop normally.

Signs and Symptoms: **Cleft lip can vary in severity and in the extent of separation seen between the lip and the nose. Cleft palate is a separation between the roof of the mouth and the nasal cavity.**

Diagnostics: Presence of abnormality.

Drug Therapy: Pain management and intravenous fluids.

Nursing Care:

Preoperatively monitor intake and output. To prevent aspiration, large nipple sizes are needed, and the infant must be fed in an upright position. Maintain a patent airway. **Keep suction at the bedside to remove excess secretions.** Teach parents proper administration of food.

Postoperatively, child restraints may be needed to prevent the infant from interfering with the incision site. A lip protector may also be placed. Infection precautions should also be maintained. After each feeding, clean the incision site each time with antibiotic ointment. For cleft palate, maintain the airway and infection precautions. Feedings are maintained, but sucking of objects is not allowed until the incision has healed. Surgery is done before the child develops teeth.

Lactose Intolerance

Definition: This is the inability to digest lactose due to a lack of the enzyme lactase in the intestines. Lactose is commonly found in dairy products.

Signs and Symptoms: Abdominal pain, diarrhea, constipation, bloating, and abdominal distension.

Diagnostics: **Hydrogen breath test.**

Drug Therapy: Enzyme medications such as Lactaid are administered. Mineral oil is given for constipation. Calcium with vitamin D is also advised.

Nursing Care: Replace dairy products with soy. A nutritionist may be consulted to speak about dietary contents. Advise the parents and the child about any age-appropriate foods that may need to be avoided.

Celiac Disease

Definition: Inability to digest gluten due to abnormal mucosa in the intestines.

Signs and Symptoms: **Foul-smelling stool, diarrhea, nausea, vomiting, irritability, anemia, and weakness.**

Complications: Celiac crisis and metabolic acidosis can occur.

Diagnostics: Stool sample and biopsy of the small intestine.

Drug Therapy: Iron, folic acid, supplements of the fat-soluble vitamins A, D, E, and K are administered.

Nursing Care: Teach the parent to avoid foods with wheat, rye, barley, and oats in the diet. Administer supplements as ordered. Monitor for celiac crisis. A nutritionist may be consulted for dietary instructions.

Failure to Thrive

Definition: This is an organic or inorganic cause of failure of a child to grow appropriately. Organic causes are drug/alcohol abuse, poverty, single parenthood, and disturbance in the mother–child bond. Common inorganic causes are AIDS, chronic renal failure, neurological imbalances, congenital heart defects, Down syndrome, and cystic fibrosis.

Signs and Symptoms: Weight loss, growth impairment, anorexia, irritability, loss of appetite, and flat affect.

Complications: Severe weight loss and malnutrition can occur.

Diagnostics: CBC and electrolytes can determine malnutrition.

Drug Therapy: Parenteral nutrition, increased calories, and IV fluids are administered.

Nursing Care: Gastric feedings may be needed in severe cases. Daily weights are done in the morning. IV fluids are administered to maintain hydration. Teach parents the importance of increasing calorie intake. Support for the family is also needed.

GENITOURINARY DISORDERS

Urinary Tract Infection

→ *Definition:* **This is an infection of the urinary tract nearly always caused by the bacterial agent *E. coli.* Girls tend to have more UTIs because of a shortened urethra.**

Signs and Symptoms: Frequent urination, incontinence, smelly urine, poor feeding, abdominal cramping, nausea, dehydration, burning during urination, diaper rash, fever, blood in urine, and excessive thirst.

Complications: Kidney infection, seizures and vesicoureteral reflux can occur.

Diagnostics: WBC, urinalysis, or dipstick of urine culture.

Drug Therapy: Antibiotics, antipyretics, and pain management.

Nursing Interventions: Monitor intake and output. Check diapers, assessing them by weight for accurate output. Administer antibiotics as ordered. Monitor temperature and signs of infection. Cranberry juice can be given to help treat symptoms. Maintain hydration and increase fluids.

Nephrotic Syndrome

Definition: This is loss of urinary protein caused by damage to the glomerulus.

Signs and Symptoms: **Four hallmark symptoms are proteinuria, hypoalbuminemia, hyperlipidemia, and edema.** Other symptoms are hypovolemia, weight gain, ascites, decreased urine output, facial edema, fatigue, and irritability. ←

Diagnostics: Electrolytes, serum albumin, protein levels, platelets, and lipid profile are commonly evaluated.

Complications: Progressive damage to the nephrons can occur if left untreated.

Drug Therapy: **High doses of corticosteroids, diuretics, and immunosuppressants are administered.** ←

Nursing Care: Monitor vital signs, intake, output, and weight. Administer medications as ordered. Steroids can cause growth retardation in children. Monitor labs during treatment. Monitor for infection and complications. Encourage fluids, and decrease sodium in the diet.

Acute Glomerulonephritis

Definition: This is inflammation of the glomeruli of the kidneys, which most often occurs after a beta-hemolytic streptococcal infection. A decrease in kidney function occurs.

Signs and Symptoms: **Periorbital edema, oliguria, tea-colored urine, acute hypertension, hematuria (grossly bloody urine), proteinuria, abdominal pain, weight loss, headache, vomiting, fever, and hypervolemia.** ←

Diagnostics: Urinalysis, BUN, creatinine, chest x-ray, urine cultures, antistreptolysin O titer to test for streptococcal infection, and renal biopsy can diagnose this disorder.

Complications: Renal failure, seizures, and heart failure can occur if left untreated.

Drug Therapy: Antihypertensives, diuretics, and antibiotics are given.

Nursing Care: Monitor blood pressure frequently, treating increased blood pressures with antihypertensive medications. Maintain fluid restriction, reducing sodium and potassium in the diet. Administer medications as ordered. Daily weights, intake, and output are obtained and recorded. Monitor for complications and CNS changes. Maintain seizure precautions. Bed rest is required during acute stages. Family teaching is needed for home care instructions.

Hemolytic Uremic Syndrome (HUS)

Definition: This is an acute renal disease that occurs after an infection caused by the bacteria *E. coli*. Hemolytic uremic syndrome is the main cause of acute renal failure in children.

Signs and Symptoms: Abdominal pain, vomiting, bloody diarrhea, bruising, oliguria, irritability, and anemia.

Diagnostics: Labs such as BUN, creatinine, hemoglobin, and hematocrit. BUN/Cr is often elevated. The H&H is often decreased to due blood loss.

Complications: Seizures and coma can occur if left untreated.

Drug Therapy: Blood transfusion and hemodialysis are used to treat this disorder.

Nursing Care: Monitor labs, vital signs, intake, and output. The child will need to have an AV shunt placed in order to receive hemodialysis. Hemodialysis care is needed. If the hemoglobin or hematocrit level is decreased, a blood transfusion is needed. Consents will need to be signed by the parents in this case. Teach the family about the disease process and treatments.

Hydrocele/Inguinal Hernia

Definition: Hydrocele is painless swelling of the scrotum caused by increased fluid and edema. Inguinal hernia is common in boys.

Signs and Symptoms: Painless swelling and edema of the scrotum and inguinal region.

Diagnostics: Clinical symptoms are used to diagnose this disorder.

Nursing Care: Prepare the patient and family for surgery. Preoperative measures are needed. Postoperatively assess the incision site and keep dressing clean. Change dressing as ordered. The child is restricted from taking any baths, and bed rest is needed.

Cryptorchidism

Definition: **Occurs when the testes fail to descend into the scrotal sac. The testes commonly descend into the scrotum by the 7th or 9th month.** Hernia can occur if left untreated.

Signs and Symptoms: Unable to feel testes in the scrotal area during assessment.

Diagnostics: Clinical symptoms are used for diagnosis. During assessment, make sure the room is warm, and the child is calm. CT/MRI can be used.

Drug Therapy: Human chorionic gonadotropin (HCG) is administered to increase testosterone levels.

Nursing Care: If the testes do not descend, a surgical procedure is done before the age of 2 years. An orchiopexy is performed to surgically descend the testes. Postoperatively monitor incision site for bleeding. Maintain infection precautions. Monitor for inguinal hernia since it is common when cryptorchidism occurs. Administer IVF and pain medications. Family education is needed for postoperative care.

Epispadias

Definition: The opening of the urethra is in the dorsal position of the penis. **Epispadias is commonly associated with bladder exstrophy.**

Signs and Symptoms: Urethral opening in the dorsal position of the penis is seen.

Diagnostics: Assessment and ultrasound can diagnose this condition.

Complications: Meatal stenosis can occur.

Drug Therapy: Oxybutynin (Ditropan) can be administered postoperatively for bladder spasms. Antibiotics are administered.

Nursing Care: Surgery is usually done for correction between the ages of 6 and 12 months. Preoperatively prepare the child and family for surgery. Postoperatively, antibiotics and pain medication are administered. Assess incision and change dressing if needed. Increase IV fluids while monitoring intake and output. **Keep activity to a minimum. The child may be placed in Bryant's traction.** Circumcision is not allowed with this condition.

Hypospadias

Definition: A urethral opening is present on the ventral side of the penis. A downward curvature of the penis may also be seen.

Signs and Symptoms: Urethral opening in the ventral region of the penis is seen.

Diagnostics: MRI/CT scan is performed.

Complications: Urinary stent or obstruction can occur postoperatively.

Nursing Care: Surgery is often performed to correct the condition. Preoperative teaching is needed. Postoperatively, antibiotics and pain management are needed. Monitor urine output; if the child is not voiding, the physician must be called, because this may indicate an obstruction. Activity is restricted, and tub baths are contraindicated until the incision is healed.

MUSCULOSKELETAL DISORDERS

Dysplasia of the Hip

Definition: Dysplasia of the hip occurs when the head of the femur is shifted or dislocated from the hip. It may occur when the infant is delivered in the breech position or when the infant is large for gestational age.

➔ *Signs and Symptoms:* **Shortening of the leg on the affected side, positive Ortolani and Barlow signs, asymmetry of the gluteal folds and the greater trochanter are seen.**

Diagnostics: MRI, x-ray, or ultrasound reveals dislocation of the hips.

Complications: If dysplasia of the hip is left untreated, it can result in impaired ambulation and limited range of motion as the child gets older.

Drug Therapy: Pain management for discomfort.

➔ *Nursing Care:* **Newborns with this disorder are placed in a Pavlik harness to maintain flexion and abduction of the hip, until the hip is in its correct form.** The harness is not removed for the first couple of weeks and, due to rapid growth, needs to be adjusted frequently as the infant grows. The infant is allowed to be out of the harness for an hour a day with the proper support of the hips. Teach parents proper diaper changing techniques, skin care, feeding, and comfort measures for the infant. Older children may need traction to correct the hip. The child is either hospitalized or meets with the physician on a weekly basis.

Congenital Clubfoot

Definition: Malformation of the foot and ankle. The most common type is talipes equinovarus, where plantar flexion is seen.

Signs and Symptoms: Malformation of the feet is the common sign.

Diagnostics: Ultrasound is performed at birth.

Drug Therapy: Pain management for discomfort or pain.

Nursing Care:

Manipulation and casting is done immediately after birth. Casting is repeated every week due to the changes in growth, until correction is seen. If there is no correction by 6 to 12 weeks, then surgical repositioning is needed. Preoperative and postoperative measures and teaching will be needed.

Cast care is important. Monitor neurovascular checks frequently. Frequent visits to the physician's office will be needed for casting. Keep the cast dry, and maintain comfort for the child. ←

Scoliosis

Definition: Lateral curvature of the spine occurs, creating an S or C shape. Scoliosis is commonly seen in preadolescent children.

Signs and Symptoms: Assessment of the spine shows curvature. Asymmetry of the ribs and flanks is seen, and the shoulder and hip are asymmetric.

Diagnostics: **The Adams test is performed by asking the child to bend over, assessing the spine for curvature.** ← Along with the Adams test, a scoliometer is used. X-rays and MRIs are done to confirm the diagnosis.

Complications: If surgery is performed, hypotension, wound infections, and delayed neurological function can occur.

Drug Therapy: Pain management is needed for discomfort and pain. If surgery is needed, pain medications and antibiotics are needed.

Nursing Care:

Patient and parent teaching are necessary before any interventions take place. A brace is the treatment of choice. **A Boston brace or thoracolumbosacral orthosis (TLSO brace) is needed.** ← The brace is worn 23 hours of the day. Monitor the skin, and teach the patient to avoid lotions and powders. Every 4 to 6 months, an x-ray is done on the spine. Body image disturbance may occur, and emotional support is needed for the patient.

If severe curvature of the spine occurs, surgery may be needed to realign the spine. Prepare the child and parents for surgery. Postoperatively monitor vital signs, neurovascular status, and incision site frequently. Monitor labs, such as hemoglobin, hematocrit, and WBC. A blood transfusion may be needed for low blood levels and blood loss during surgery. Pain management is based on the individual and administered as ordered. Maintain alignment and logroll the patient when needed.

Juvenile Idiopathic Arthritis

Definition: This is an autoimmune inflammatory disease of the joints.

Signs and Symptoms: Joint pain, swelling, and limited range of motion are seen.

Diagnostics: X-rays and increased erythrocyte sedimentation rate levels.

Complications: Disability and acute uveitis can cause blindness.

Drug Therapy: NSAIDs, methotrexate, corticosteroids, and slow-acting antirheumatic drugs (SAARDs) are administered.

Nursing Care: Treat each symptom individually. Administer medications as ordered. Maintain proper pain management. Regular eye exams are done routinely. Assess joint for swelling or tenderness. Hot and cold therapy can decrease discomfort. Physical therapy is needed. Provide emotional support.

Duchenne Muscular Dystrophy (DMD)

Definition: Pseudohypertrophic (Duchenne) muscular dystrophy is the most common muscular dystrophy disorder in children. **DMD is caused by an absence of the protein dystrophin, which results from a genetic defect on the X chromosome.**

Signs and Symptoms: Unsteady gait, falls easily, hip/knee contractures, scoliosis, postural changes, cognitive difficulty, obesity, muscles enlarged on the thighs and upper arms, and weakened calf muscles.

→ *Diagnostics:* **Muscle biopsy, electromyography (EMG), DNA testing, and serum creatine kinase (CK) is elevated.**

Complications: Cardiac and respiratory failure can occur if left untreated.

Drug Therapy: Prednisone can be used to decrease loss of muscle function.

Nursing Care: There is no cure for DMD. The main intervention is to maintain ambulation and range of motion. To maintain muscle function braces, physical therapy, weight control, and stretching exercises are helpful. Maintain a safe environment for the child since falling occurs frequently. Maintain respiratory function by using an incentive spirometer. Family and patient support is needed.

HEMATOLOGICAL DISORDERS

Iron Deficiency Anemia

Definition: Iron (Fe) is needed for hemoglobin production. When there is a lack of iron (e.g., because of insufficient dietary iron or pregnancy), iron deficiency anemia as well as a decrease in hemoglobin results.

Sign and Symptoms: **Pallor, fatigue, poor muscle tone, and irritability.** ←

Diagnostics: Labs such as hemoglobin levels, serum Fe, and presence of reticulocytes.

Complications: Infection, cardiac dysfunction, and hypoxemia can occur in severe cases.

Drug Therapy: Iron is given orally and by the intramuscular route.

Nursing Care: Increase iron intake orally through formula. For toddlers, give iron-rich foods such as bread, cereal, whole grains, raisins, and meats. Teach the parents to give iron supplements on an empty stomach. If iron is mixed with juice, it should be given with a straw to prevent staining of the teeth. If injection Fe is given, do not massage site and assess for allergic reactions. Iron can cause constipation, and parents should assess for this side effect. Iron levels will be retested in 3 months.

Sickle Cell Anemia

Definition: This is **a hereditary autosomal recessive disorder. Hemoglobin A cells are replaced by sickle hemoglobin**. Red blood cells are obstructed and ischemic due to the sickle hemoglobin. Infection, pain, and stress can cause cells to sickle. ←

Signs and Symptoms: Symptoms are based on the particular crisis that can occur. Fever, hypoxemia, increased hemoglobin, and dehydration can cause a crisis. **The two main types are vaso-occlusive and sequestration crisis. Symptoms of vaso-occlusive crisis are fever, swelling of joints, bone pain, abdominal pain, frontal bossing, visual changes, jaundice, and priapism. Symptoms of sequestration crisis are hypovolemia, pallor, weakness, increased heart rate, hypotension, dyspnea, and abdominal distension.** ←

Diagnostics: Labs such as hemoglobin, hematocrit, reticulocytes, and sickle-turbidity test are performed.

Complications: Acute chest syndrome, CVA, cardiomegaly, renal failure, seizures, blindness, liver cirrhosis, and splenomegaly can occur.

Drug Therapy: Opioids are given for pain; antibiotics, immunizations, corticosteroids, and analgesics are also given.

Nursing Care: Administering oxygen and maintaining hydration can decrease crisis occurrence. Blood transfusions are given to increase perfusion. The child remains on bed rest to conserve energy. Administer pain medications as ordered. Monitor for complications. Reduce the risk of infections through antibiotics and immunizations. Teach parents to assess for complications and report to the physician immediately.

Beta-Thalassemia (Cooley Anemia)

Definition: This is an autosomal recessive disorder that causes a deficiency in hemoglobin levels, resulting in severe anemia.

→ *Signs and Symptoms:* **Pallor, fatigue, increased bilirubin, weight loss, enlarged spleen, headache, frontal bossing, flattened nose, and anemia.**

Diagnostics: Labs such as hemoglobin and hematocrit show anemia. Hemoglobin electrophoresis is used to diagnose the patient.

Complications: Organ failure and heart disease can occur from increased iron production.

Drug Therapy: Blood transfusions are done frequently. To treat iron overload, chelation therapy with deferoxamine (Desferal) is given to prevent organ damage.

Nursing Care: Administer blood transfusion to maintain healthy blood levels. → **Chelation therapy is administered to prevent organ damage.** Due to frequent transfusions, the child may develop splenomegaly and may require a splenectomy. Parent teaching is needed, and monitoring for complications is key.

Von Willebrand Disease

→ *Definition:* This is **a hereditary bleeding disorder that causes prolonged bleeding time and decreased levels of factor VIII.**

Signs and Symptoms: Bruising, nosebleeds, and excessive menstrual bleeding.

Diagnostics: Labs such as platelets and blood levels are used for diagnosis.

Complications: Excessive bleeding can cause severe anemia.

Drug Therapy: **Desmopressin acetate (DDAVP) is given along with the administration of factor VIII.** ←

Nursing Care: Monitor labs and assess for bleeding. Administer medication as ordered. Avoid aspirin since it can cause bleeding. Patient teaching is needed for episodes of bleeding. Blood transfusion may be needed based on blood levels.

Hemophilia

Definition: This is an X-linked recessive disorder. Hemophilia is a group of bleeding disorders that results in a lack of ability to coagulate the blood. The most common type is factor VIII deficiency.

Signs and Symptoms: Bruises easily, hematuria, bleeding occurs in joints (hemarthrosis), and intracranial hemorrhage and anemia can occur.

Diagnostics: Labs such as PTT and low levels of factor VIII are seen.

Complications: Intracranial hemorrhage and bleeding in the throat can cause airway obstruction, and hematomas in the spine can cause paralysis.

Drug Therapy: Factor VIII, DDAVP, and corticosteroids are administered.

Nursing Care: Monitor for bleedings, and maintain precautions to decrease risk of bleeding. Administer medications as needed. Use a soft toothbrush to decrease bleeding from the gums. The child's school should be aware of the disorder. Avoid aspirin since it can cause bleeding. Monitor joint pain and bleeding by immobilizing, resting the joint, applying ice, and elevating the extremity. Parents are taught the measures to take if bleeding occurs at home.

PEDIATRIC CANCERS

Neuroblastoma

Definition: This is an extracranial nonlymphatic tumor. It is the most common type of tumor in children and is known as the "silent tumor" due to asymptomatic manifestations. A common finding is an abdominal tumor.

Signs and Symptoms: The abdomen has a palpable mass. Urinary retention, hypertension, increased heart rate, bone pain, edema, weight loss, vomiting, nausea, and generalized weakness are common symptoms.

Diagnostics: Bone scans, biopsy of the mass, and bone marrow aspiration are performed.

Complications: Further tumor progression can occur if not treated.

Drug Therapy: Radiation, chemotherapy, antiemetic, pain management, and total parenteral nutrition may be administered.

Nursing Care: Administer chemotherapy and radiation as prescribed. Teach the parents the treatment plan and goals. If the child has to undergo surgery, preoperative and postoperative teaching is necessary. Monitor for complications. Maintain good nutrition and hydration. Maintain intake, output, and vital signs per protocol.

Wilm's Tumor

Definition: This is the most common type of renal cancer in children.

Signs and Symptoms: Abdominal mass, nausea, vomiting, abdominal pain, anemia, hematuria, hypertension, and abdominal distension.

Diagnostics: Do not palpate the mass due to risk of rupturing. An ultrasound of the abdomen can detect mass.

Complications: Further progression of tumor staging.

Drug Therapy: Radiation, chemotherapy, and pain management are often prescribed.

Nursing Care: A nephrectomy of the kidney may be needed. Administer chemotherapy or radiation as prescribed. Preoperative, postoperative, and medication teaching are needed for both parent and child. Maintain intake, output, and vital signs. Monitor for complications.

Osteogenic Sarcoma

Definition: This is the most common type of bone cancer in children. The most common tumor site is the femur.

Signs and Symptoms: Palpable mass on the femur, nausea, vomiting, and pain at the site.

Diagnostics: CT scan can detect mass.

Complications: Further progression of tumor.

Drug Therapy: Chemotherapy, antiemetic, and pain management are often administered.

Nursing Care: Surgery is often needed if the tumor is not treated with chemotherapy. Medication treatment and teaching are necessary. Maintain hydration and nutrition. Monitor for complications.

Acute Lymphocytic Leukemia (ALL)

Definition: This is a malignant disorder caused by immature lymphoid cells called lymphoblasts. It is commonly found outside the blood or bone marrow.

Signs and Symptoms: Anemia, infection, bleeding, fever, pallor, bruising, bone pain, irritability, GI upset, headache, nuchal rigidity, splenomegaly, and hepatomegaly.

Diagnostics: Lumbar puncture, bone marrow aspiration, chest x-ray, and examination of CSF. Abnormal labs such as increased leukocyte, decreased hemoglobin, and decreased platelets can confirm the diagnosis.

Complications: Bleeding, increased intracranial pressure, and infection can occur.

Drug Therapy: Chemotherapy, antiemetics, and antibiotics are administered.

Nursing Care: Monitor vital signs and labs. Administer intrathecal chemotherapy as ordered. Monitor for infection and bleeding. Provide small meals, and encourage child to conserve energy for feedings. Provide adequate hydration. Monitor for complications, and report to the physician immediately if there is occurrence. Due to the side effects of chemotherapy, hair loss and GI upset may occur. Teach parents that these are temporary side effects of the chemotherapy. Administer medications to treat GI side effects.

Acute Myelogenous Leukemia (AML)

Definition: Bone marrow failure occurs due to a decrease in bone marrow cells. AML is caused by exposure to chemicals, cigarette smoke, and drugs used in utero.

Signs and Symptoms: Anemia, thrombocytopenia, and neutropenia.

Diagnostics: Bone marrow aspiration is the definitive test.

Complications: Hemorrhagic cystitis, infection, bleeding, and gingival hyperplasia.

Drug Therapy: Chemotherapy and antiemetics are administered.

Nursing Care: Administer chemotherapy as ordered. Teach the parents side effects of this therapy before administering doses. GI upset may occur; administer antiemetics to decrease side effects. Assess for gingival hyperplasia. Use soft toothbrush, and provide oral care to decrease risk. Alopecia may occur; reassure parents that regrowth is common. Provide adequate nutrition and maintain hydration. Emotional support is needed. Provide information on support groups.

EAR, EYE, AND THROAT DISORDERS

Conjunctivitis

Definition: This is inflammation of the conjunctiva, which is also known as "pinkeye." It is caused by infection or allergies.

Signs and Symptoms: Itching, burning, redness, swelling, and a white discharge from the eye are seen.

Diagnostics: Diagnosis is based on the presence of symptoms.

Drug Therapy: Antibiotics are administered directly to the eye, and antihistamines may be given.

Nursing Care: Prevent infection and transmission to the eye by using separate towels and proper hand-washing techniques. Administer medications as ordered. Teach the parents and child to avoid rubbing the infected eye. To decrease swelling and discomfort, cold compresses can be applied to the eyes.

Otitis Media

Definition: This is an inflammatory disorder of the middle ear.

Signs and Symptoms: Fever, earache, ear drainage, reddened tympanic membrane, and irritability can occur.

Diagnostics: Otoscopic assessment of the tympanic membrane.

→ **When assessing the tympanic membrane in children 3 years or younger, pull the ear lobe down and back. In children older than 3, including adults, pull the pinna up and back.**

Drug Therapy: Antibiotics, antipyretics, and analgesics are administered.

Nursing Care: Administer medication as ordered. Monitor for discomfort, and administer medication as ordered. If ear infections recur, a myringotomy may need to be performed. A myringotomy is the insertion of tympanoplasty tubes in the middle ear to maintain equal pressure. Postoperatively administer pain medications as ordered. Ear plugs should be worn when bathing or swimming. If the myringotomy tube falls out, this is not considered a medical emergency, and the physician should be called. **Avoid blowing the child's nose postoperatively.** ←

Tonsillectomy and Adenoidectomy

Definition: Inflammation of the tonsils and adenoids.

Signs and Symptoms: Sore throat, redness, bad breath, white patches on the throat, fever, and difficulty swallowing.

Diagnostics: Assessment of symptoms confirms diagnosis.

Complications: Hemorrhage can occur postoperatively.

Drug Therapy: Antibiotics and pain management are administered.

Nursing Care: Prepare the child and family for surgery. Preoperatively monitor labs and vital signs, and assess for any loose teeth. Postoperatively monitor vital signs, administer medications as ordered, maintain a side-lying position, and provide a clear liquid diet. **Teach the parents and child to avoid any red liquid and the use of straws.** ← Assess for complications such as hemorrhage.

INFECTIOUS DISORDERS

Chickenpox (Varicella)

Definition: This is caused by the varicella-zoster virus (VZV). It is transmitted through direct contact, droplets, and contaminated items. The virus can be spread from 1 to 2 days before the onset of the rash until the sixth day, when the lesions or rash have dried. The incubation period is usually 2 to 3 weeks.

Signs and Symptoms: Fever and loss of appetite; a macular rash appears on all the extremities, abdomen, face, scalp, and genital areas.

Diagnostics: Based on the presentation of symptoms.

Complications: Pneumonia, encephalitis, and hemorrhagic varicella can occur.

Drug Therapy: Calamine lotion is applied to the skin. Antibiotics are administered.

Nursing Care: Contact and droplet precautions are maintained throughout the hospital and in the home, especially during the communicable period. Administer calamine lotion to the skin; parents should wear gloves while applying this. Cool baths can help decrease the discomfort. The child can return to school when the lesions have crusted.

Measles (Rubeola)

Definition: Measles is transmitted through contact and droplets. The virus can be spread from 4 days before to 5 days after the appearance of the rash. The incubation period is 10 to 20 days.

Signs and Symptoms: Fever, cough, and photophobia; maculopapular rash appears on the body, and Koplik's spots (red spots with a bluish white center) are seen on the buccal mucosa.

Diagnostics: Based on the presentation of symptoms.

Complications: Pneumonia and encephalitis can occur.

Drug Therapy: Antipyretics and antibiotics are administered.

Nursing Care: Droplet and contact precautions are maintained in the hospital until the fifth day of the rash. Maintain skin care, and teach the parent to keep the skin dry and clean. The child is placed on bed rest with minimum activity. To treat photophobia, lights should be kept dim. Administer antipyretics to treat fever.

Mumps

Definition: Mumps is transmitted through contact and droplets. It is most commonly spread through saliva. Mumps can spread immediately upon contact. The incubation period is 14 to 21 days.

Signs and Symptom: Headache, fever, loss of appetite, earache, and parotid gland swelling are common symptoms.

Diagnostics: Based on the presentation of symptoms.

Complications: Encephalitis, arthritis, and hepatitis could occur.

Drug Therapy: Antipyretics, analgesics, and antibiotics are administered.

Nursing Care: Isolation precautions are needed. Administer analgesics if the child experiences pain. Antipyretics are used to treat a fever. Soups are recommended during this time because chewing increases pain. Hot and cold compresses are applied to the neck to relieve discomfort.

Roseola (Exanthema Subitum)

Definition: This is caused by the human herpesvirus type 6 (HHV-6). The route of transmission is unknown. The incubation period is 5 to 15 days.

Signs and Symptoms: Fever is the main symptom, along with the appearance of pink macular rash on the body.

Diagnostics: Based on the presentation of symptoms.

Complications: Seizures and encephalitis can occur.

Drug Therapy: Antipyretics, antibiotics, and anticonvulsants are administered.

Nursing Care: Administer antipyretics for fever. Maintain seizure precautions. Monitor for complications.

Fifth Disease (Erythema Infectiosum)

Definition: This is caused by human parvovirus B19 (HPV). It is transmitted through respiratory droplets and blood. The incubation period is 4 to 20 days.

Signs and Symptoms: Fever and headache are the main symptoms, rash appears as "slapped cheek," and maculopapular red rash occurs on the body.

Diagnostics: Based on the presentation of symptoms.

Complications: Arthritis and fetal death can occur if a woman is infected during pregnancy.

Drug Therapy: Antipyretics, analgesics, and anti-inflammatory medications are administered.

Nursing Care: Isolation is not needed for the patients. Home care with medication administration treats this disease. Pregnant women should avoid children with fifth disease due to increased risk of complications.

Diphtheria

Definition: This is caused by *Corynebacterium diphtheria*. It is transmitted through contact with the carrier. The incubation period is 2 to 5 days.

Signs and Symptoms: **Fever; sore throat; nasal drainage; neck edema, which produces a "bull neck" appearance; and cough.** ←

Diagnostics: **Based on the presentation of symptoms.** ←

Complications: Airway obstruction, cyanosis, and myocarditis can occur.

Drug Therapy: Antitoxin (to rule out sensitivity to horse serum), antipyretics, and antibiotics are administered.

Nursing Care: Isolation precautions are needed. Maintain a patent airway. Keep a tracheostomy and suction kit at the bedside. Administer medications as ordered. Administer oxygen as needed. Monitor vital signs. The child is maintained on bed rest with minimum activity.

Rocky Mountain Spotted Fever

Definition: This is caused by *Rickettsia rickettsii* and transmitted through a tick bite. The incubation period is 2 to 14 days.

Signs and Symptoms: Fever, headache, GI upset, and maculopapular rash on extremities.

Diagnostics: Based on the presentation of symptoms.

Drug Therapy: Antibiotics and antipyretics.

Nursing Care: Administer medications as ordered. Teach parent and child the preventive measures to avoid tick bites.

Whooping Cough (Pertussis)

Definition: This is caused by *Bordetella pertussis*. It is transmitted through contact and respiratory droplets. The incubation period is 5 to 20 days.

Signs and Symptoms: Fever, dry hacking cough that sounds like a "whoop," and increased respiratory secretions.

Diagnostics: Based on the presentation of symptoms.

Complications: Pneumonia, seizures, and otitis media.

Drug Therapy: Administer antimicrobials such as erythromycin, pertussis immune globulin, and antipyretics as ordered.

Nursing Care: Contact precautions are initiated. Monitor respiratory status, and apply oxygen as needed. Monitor vital signs. Administer medications as ordered. Teach the child and the parent to avoid places with smoke or dust. Home care involves parents assessing child respiratory status and monitoring for complications.

Scarlet Fever

→ *Definition:* This is caused by **group A beta-hemolytic streptococci.** It is transmitted through direct contact of carrier or droplets. It is contagious for the first 2 weeks of diagnosis. The incubation period is 1 to 7 days.

Signs and Symptoms: Fever, headache, abdominal pain, GI upset, sandpaper-like rash, **strawberry-like tongue,** edematous tonsils and pharynx. Rash is present on the joints, and desquamation of the skin occurs. ←

Diagnostics: Based on the presentation of symptoms.

Complications: Glomerulonephritis and otitis media.

Drug Therapy: Antibiotics such as penicillin are used.

Nursing Care: Respiratory precautions are initiated until antibiotic therapy begins. The child is put on bed rest with minimum activity. Administer medications as ordered. Maintain hydration.

Infectious Mononucleosis

Definition: This is caused by the Epstein–Barr virus and transmitted through oral secretions. The incubation period is 4 to 6 weeks.

Signs and Symptoms: Fever, headache, cough, sore throat, GI upset, and edematous tonsils.

Diagnostics: Based on the presentation of symptoms.

Complications: Lymphadenopathy and hepatosplenomegaly.

Drug Therapy: Antibiotics and antipyretics are administered.

Nursing Care: Avoid contact sports during this period in view of the complication of rupturing of the spleen. Teach the patient and the child to monitor for complications. Administer medications as ordered.

IMMUNIZATIONS

Sorry to break the bad news, but you will have to know the recommended immunizations for both children and adolescents. Go to the Centers for Disease Control website, and print the most current immunizations for the year. Before administration of any immunization, it is important to provide parents with all the information, including side effects. After administration, assess for soreness and redness at the site. The professors will test you on the vaccinations needed for each age group. Be familiar with any new vaccines.

SEVEN

WOMEN'S HEALTH

Welcome to women's health. This is where it all begins. This is where you will experience firsthand the journey between preconception and birth. This course is usually taken with a pediatric nursing course because they pretty much go hand in hand. You will need to know the developmental stages a family experiences during the childbearing process, along with any complications that may occur in the prenatal, intrapartum, and postpartum stages.

The clinical portion of this course will help you tremendously in mastering this information. You will be able to practice nursing care of women in all stages from the prenatal to labor and delivery. In the labor and delivery unit, you will experience the end stages of labor to the birth of the newborn. You will be able to be part of the experience of both a vaginal and a cesarean birth. In the postpartum unit, you will be able to perform a full assessment on the newborn.

You will also experience the neonatal intensive care unit (NICU). Infants in the NICU require close monitoring, feedings, respiratory support, and intravenous therapy. During my clinical experience, I was able to monitor an infant born with trisomy 18, which is a syndrome with deformities that are incompatible with life. It was emotionally difficult to witness, but I quickly realized that, in this profession, both life and death must be faced. Family support and emotional support are very important during difficult times. On the other hand, it is always amazing to see patients who are critically ill become well and strong again.

The exams in this course do mimic the stages of birth. There are not too many disorders to remember, and most exam questions were based on the various stages and manifestations that both infant and mother experience. The clinical portion will be based on your ability to assess a mother and a newborn and to identify the complications that could arise. This was a very enjoyable course for me, and I hope that you have the same experience. As a mother, I know the joyous moments that occurred during these stages. You will be able to experience and share the same moments with families during clinical.

FETAL DEVELOPMENT

Embryonic Stage

The embryonic stage begins 3 weeks after conception and lasts until the 8th week of gestation.

- 3rd week: The heart, arm, and leg buds are formed.
- 4th week: Eyes, nose, heart, and gastrointestinal tract develop.
- 6th week: Abdominal trunk, fingers, liver, and trachea are formed.
- 8th week: The embryonic stage ends in the 8th week, during which time the muscles, ears, fingers, and toes are developed.

Fetal Stage

The fetal stage is between week 8 and the end of pregnancy.

- 12 weeks: The eyelids are prominent, the fetal heartbeat can be heard, gender can be determined, and movement occurs.
- 16 weeks: Fine hair, blood vessels, teeth and kidneys are formed, and meconium production occurs.
- 20 weeks: The spinal cord begins to develop, quickening (fetal movement) is felt by a first-time mother, and brown fat appears.
- 24 weeks: The fetus responds to sound, opens eyes, and makes a fist; alveoli on the lungs form; and the body is covered with vernix caseosa (thick white covering).
- 28 weeks: The brain is developing, the nervous system develops, the lungs are able to breathe in air, but the major organs are still immature for birth.
- 36 weeks: Skin appears pink, and fingers and toenails are fully developed.
- 38 to 40 weeks: The mother is preparing for the birth of the infant, and the fetus is considered full term. If labor occurs at 37 weeks or less, it is considered a preterm delivery.

THE PRENATAL EXPERIENCE

Stages of Labor

Antepartum: The time between conception and onset of labor.

Intrapartum: Onset of labor until the birth of the infant and the delivery of placenta occur.

Postpartum: After the birth of the newborn up to the return of the woman's recovery; the typical recovery time is 6 weeks.

Determination of Due Date and the Acronym GTPAL

Nagele's Rule is used to determine the woman's due date based on the 28-day menstrual cycle. To estimate the due date, count back 3 months, add 7 days, and change the year.

GTPAL is used to determine the woman's past pregnancy history. **G** refers to *gravidity,* which is the number of pregnancies, including the present one. **T** is the number of pregnancies brought to *term* beyond 37 weeks of gestation. **P** is the number of pregnancies delivered born *preterm* before 37 weeks of gestation. **A** refers to the number of spontaneous or therapeutic *abortions* that occurred. **L** refers to the number of *living* children that the woman has given birth to.

Signs of Pregnancy

Presumptive Signs: Nausea, vomiting, quickening, breast tenderness, fatigue, vaginal changes, amenorrhea, and urinary frequency occur. This may also be mistaken for menstrual cycle symptoms.

Probable Signs: Goodell's sign—softening of the cervix; Chadwick's sign—bluish discoloration of vaginal secretions; Hegar's sign—thinning of the uterine wall; and Braxton Hicks contractions (false labor pain).

Positive Signs: Fetal heart sounds and movement felt by examiner, or diagnostic confirmation of a fetus, which is detected through an ultrasound or examination.

Laboratory and Diagnostic Tests

Laboratory Tests

These include a Pap smear, CBC, hemoglobin, rubella titer, ABO and Rh typing, glucose levels, hepatitis B screen, sexually transmitted infection (STI), sickle cell screen, tuberculin skin test, and urinalysis with culture, which are done prenatally and throughout the pregnancy.

Diagnostic Tests

Quad Screen: A screening done between 16 and 18 weeks of pregnancy to assess for neural tube defects such as trisomies 21 and 18.

Chorionic Villus Sampling (CVS): Aspiration of the chorionic villi from the placenta to detect any genetic abnormalities. CVS is performed at 8 to 12 weeks of gestation.

Fetal Biophysical Profile (BBP): Assesses fetal well-being based on five criteria: fetal breathing movements, body movements, muscle tone, nonstress test, and amniotic fluid volume.

Maternal Nutrition

Prenatal vitamins are prescribed, which include folic acid. Folic acid deficiency can cause disorders such as spina bifida. Ferrous sulfate (Fe) is administered if the patient experiences anemia, with frequent monitoring of blood levels. Teach the mother to maintain a healthy, balanced diet throughout the pregnancy. Decrease foods that might cause nausea or heartburn. Antacids can be given before meals to treat heartburn.

The Complicated Prenatal Experience

Abortion

Definition: A pregnancy that either ends spontaneously or is voluntarily terminated before 20 weeks of gestation.

Side Effects: Vaginal bleeding, hemorrhage, shock, and contractions can occur.

Nursing Care: Monitor vital signs and amount of vaginal bleeding. Increase fluid intake, and continue to monitor the patient for signs of shock or hemorrhage. Contraceptive teaching is needed.

Gestational Diabetes

Definition: Changes in insulin tolerance during pregnancy. The pancreas is unable to meet the increased demand for insulin production.

→ *Signs and Symptoms:* **The 3 Ps—polyuria, polydipsia, and polyphagia—are common symptoms**. Other symptoms include weight loss, blurred vision, neuritis, weakness, and hyperglycemia.

Diagnostics: 3-hour oral glucose tolerance test (GTT) and hemoglobin A1C level.

Complications: Large-for-gestational-age (LGA) fetus can occur if diabetes is left untreated.

Drug Therapy: If not controlled with diet, then insulin will be prescribed.

Nursing Care: Teach the patient to monitor diet and assess blood glucose before meals and at bedtime. Most mothers with gestational diabetes can control blood glucose levels through diet by maintaining an 1,800 calorie ADA diet. If insulin is needed, teach the patient how to use a sliding scale. Teach the patient to assess for infection, hypoglycemia, and other complications.

Pregnancy-Induced Hypertension

Definition: Gestational hypertension develops after 20 weeks and is characterized by high blood pressure and the presence of protein in the urine. Preeclampsia occurs when there is an increase in blood pressure after 20 weeks, with no prior history of hypertension. Eclampsia is the occurrence of seizures in pregnant women who suffer from preeclampsia.

Signs and Symptoms: **Hypertension, proteinuria, edema, headache, and restlessness are the hallmark symptoms.** ←

Diagnostics: BUN, creatinine, 24-hour urine levels assessing for protein, and blood pressure.

Complications: Eclampsia is seizures caused by untreated high blood pressure.

Drug Therapy: Antihypertensive medications and magnesium sulfate are administered to the patient.

Nursing Care: Maintain seizure precautions. Monitor fetal activity. Monitor blood pressure. The patient may be put on bed rest or limited activity. For women who suffer from preeclampsia, monitor for complications of the HELLP syndrome (hemolysis, elevated liver enzymes, and low platelet count). Administer antihypertensive medications as ordered. Teach the patient to monitor blood pressure and to watch for complications.

Women With HIV/AIDS

Definition: Women with HIV are at an increased risk for complications and infection. The fetus is at risk for transmission through the mother's fluids and blood.

Signs and Symptoms: Fever, sore throat, swollen lymph nodes, shingles, and fatigue. These patients are considered immunocompromised.

Diagnostics: ELISA, western blot, and IFA are done to diagnose HIV and AIDS.

Complications: Infants born small for gestational age (SGA), and transmission of the HIV infection.

Drug Therapy: Azidothymine (AZT) and zidovudine (ZDV) are administered.

Nursing Care: Prenatally monitor labs, vital signs, fetal growth, and any signs of infection. Teach the patient to avoid any procedures such as amniocentesis or fetal scalp sampling. During labor and delivery, if the fetus is not infected with HIV, minimize the infant's exposure to maternal blood or fluids. Postnatal measures are very important to prevent transmission of the disease. Newborns are given antiretroviral and continued treatments for 4 weeks. A CBC is performed to assess whether transmission of the virus occurred. Frequent visits to the physician are necessary during the first weeks of life to assess for any complications or signs of infection. Teach the mother and family the importance of administration of medication, follow-up visits, and assessing for infection.

Disseminated Intravascular Coagulation (DIC)

Definition: Decrease of platelets and clotting factors causes clots to form in the bloodstream of pregnant women. DIC can be caused by prenatal complications such as gestational diabetes or fetal death.

Signs and Symptoms: Excessive bleeding, bruising, hematuria, weakness, pallor, and blood in the stool.

Diagnostics: Labs such as PT, PTT, INR, platelets, fibrinogen, platelets, and hematocrit are monitored.

Complications: Shock can occur from blood loss.

Drug Therapy: Blood transfusion may be needed, heparin may be prescribed, and IV fluids are needed.

Nursing Care: Monitor labs, vital signs, fetal growth and activity. Administer medications as ordered. If a transfusion is needed, obtain consents and continue to monitor labs. Monitor intake and output. Monitor for complications such as shock.

Iron Deficiency Anemia/Folic Acid Deficiency Anemia

Definition: Iron deficiency anemia occurs when there is a decrease in serum ferritin levels due to the increased iron demands during pregnancy. Folic acid deficiency anemia occurs when there is a decrease in serum folate levels due to inadequate intake of folic acid.

Signs and Symptoms: Weakness, pallor, headache, and decreased blood levels occur in iron deficiency anemia. Symptoms of folic acid deficiency are nausea, vomiting, and weight loss.

Diagnostics: Labs such as hemoglobin, hematocrit, ferritin, and folate levels.

Complications: **Folic acid deficiency can cause neural defects in a fetus**. Iron deficiency anemia can cause low birth weight and neonatal death.

Drug Therapy: Iron and folic acid supplements are administered.

Nursing Care: Monitor labs and fetal growth. Administer supplements as ordered. Advise on the need for increased iron and folic acid in the diet. Monitor for complications, and teach the importance of prenatal visits. Iron supplements are best given with vitamin C for absorption.

Hyperemesis Gravidarum

Definition: This refers to a change in electrolytes and nutrition due to excessive vomiting and nausea.

Signs and Symptoms: Nausea, vomiting, dehydration, electrolyte imbalances, hypotension, and weakness.

Diagnostics: Labs such as electrolytes, BUN, creatinine, and hematocrit levels.

Complications: Dehydration, hypokalemia, premature birth, and maternal death can occur.

Drug Therapy: IV fluids with potassium, corticosteroids, and antiemetics.

Nursing Care: Monitor labs, fetal activity, vital signs, and weight. Administer IV fluids and order total parenteral nutrition (TPN) to replace electrolyte imbalance. Teach the patient the importance of hydration. Monitor for weight loss and complications.

Incompetent Cervix

Definition: Premature dilation of the cervix is due to an incompetent cervix. Dilation is painless, and the patient is not aware of the premature dilation. Dilation can occur as early as 16 to 24 weeks of pregnancy.

Signs and Symptoms: Bleeding, pelvic pressure, and bulging membranes are present.

Diagnostics: Ultrasound can diagnose this disorder by identifying a short cervix or one that is opening internally.

Complications: Premature rupture of membranes.

Drug Therapy: Antibiotics are administered to decrease the risk of infection. Tocolysis is administered to decrease contractions.

Nursing Care: Ultrasound is used to diagnose incompetent cervix. Continue fetal monitoring. The patient remains on bed rest, IV fluids are administered, and medications are administered. A cervical cerclage can be performed, in which the cervix is sutured closed, and it is then removed during the 37th week of pregnancy. Home care consists of monitoring for infection and complications.

Premature Rupture of Membranes (PROM)

Definition: This refers to rupturing of membranes before the onset of labor and before 37 weeks.

Signs and Symptoms: Fluid expelled and pelvic pressure.

→ *Diagnostics:* **Nitrazine paper is used to test for the presence of amniotic fluid**; CBC, urinalysis, and ultrasound are performed.

Complications: Infection, fetal mortality, and premature birth can occur.

Drug Therapy: Antibiotics and betamethasone (Diprolene) are administered.

Nursing Care: Monitor vital signs, administer medications as prescribed, place the patient on the left side, and monitor for infections. Monitor fetal status and activity. A nonstress test may be performed to accurately assess fetal well-being. If necessary, prepare the patient for preterm labor.

LABOR AND DELIVERY

Fetal Monitoring

Leopold's Maneuvers: These maneuvers are used to evaluate fetal position and fetal heartbeats. The mother is advised to empty her bladder and lie on her back to perform the maneuvers. The first maneuver determines where the fetal head is located in the pelvis. The second maneuver palpates the fetus back and extremities. The third maneuver assesses the presenting part and the position of the fetus, either cephalic (head down) or breech (buttocks).The fourth maneuver is assessing the descent of the fetus into the pelvis.

External Fetal Monitoring: Fetal heart tones (FHTs) can be heard and identified through the mother's abdomen by using an ultrasound or Doppler device. The normal fetal heart rate (FHR) is 110 to 150 bpm. Leopold's maneuver is performed to find the position of the fetus because the FHT is best heard over the fetus's back.

Internal Fetal Monitoring: Internal fetal monitoring is done by attaching an electrode to the fetal scalp by inserting it through the vagina and cervix once the fetal membranes are ruptured. In order for internal monitoring to be performed, the cervix must be at least 3 cm dilated.

Fetal Heart Patterns

Normal Fetal Heart Rate: The normal FHR is 110 to 160 bpm. It is obtained through external or internal monitoring.

Tachycardia: In tachycardia, the FHR is more than 160 bpm. Tachycardia can result from dehydration or fever.

Bradycardia: In bradycardia, the FHT decreases to less than 110 bpm for 10 minutes or longer. Bradycardia can be caused by umbilical cord compression, hypotension, and fetal hypoxemia.

Variability: Variability describes the normal fluctuations in the baseline FHR. Decreased variability can be caused by a period of fetal rest. Increased variability can be caused by contractions or stress on the fetus.

Accelerations: An increase in the FHR that is periodic usually occur from fetal activity. Acceleration can also be caused by contractions.

Decelerations: Decelerations are a decrease in the FHR. There are three types—early, late, and variable decelerations. Early deceleration is a brief decrease in heart rate due to compression of the fetal head against the pelvis during descent. These decelerations are seen during a contraction. A variable deceleration is a decrease in heart rate due to umbilical cord compression. Variable decelerations last between 15 seconds and 2 minutes and look like a V or W on the monitor. Late decelerations are caused by uteroplacental insufficiency. Late decelerations require immediate attention because there is a lack of blood flow or oxygen to the fetus. The first nursing interactions are to reposition the mother on her side, turn off any oxytocin that may be running, and give oxygen via mask at 10 L when late decelerations are seen.

Stages of Labor

First Stage: The first stage of labor is divided into three phases: latent, active, and transition.

The latent stage is the mild contractions; cervical dilation is 1 to 3 cm. The active phase is cervical dilation of 4 to 7 cm, fetal descent begins, and contractions are more frequent and intense. In the transition phase, cervical dilation of 7 to 10 cm takes place, contractions become intense, and the patient may feel the urge to push.

Second Stage: The second stage spans the complete dilation of the cervix to the birth of the infant. The contractions are intense, the mother begins to push, and crowning occurs (fetal head is seen).

Third Stage: The third stage is the birth of the infant to the birth of the placenta separation. The placenta is usually expelled within 30 minutes after the birth of the infant.

Fourth Stage: The fourth stage is from the birth of the placenta to 2 to 4 hours after. The patient's vital signs return to normal. Involution discomfort is usually present. The mother's appetite returns, and she may request food. Pain management is needed as well.

Birth Procedures

Cervical Ripening: Cervical ripening is used to induce labor by softening the cervix. One method of aiding cervical ripening is with prostaglandin E gel. Consents are signed before the procedure. After insertion, the patient must lie supine for 1 hour. Labor may occur within 24 hours of administration. Another method of cervical ripening involves insertion of a Foley catheter into the cervix followed by inflation of a 30 mL balloon.

Labor Induction: Induction stimulates contractions to initiate labor before the presence of natural labor or rupturing of the membranes. The most common method is administration of oxytocin (Pitocin) IV to begin stimulation of contractions. Before medication administration, obtain maternal vital signs and assess the FHR. Oxytocin is started in small dosages (2 mU/minutes) until adequate labor is obtained. Once the patient begins to have consistent contractions every 2 minutes, oxytocin is discontinued.

Amniotomy: An amniotomy is artificial rupturing of the membranes to augment labor. The patient must be at least 2 cm dilated. Before the procedure, the fetal presentation, station, position, and FHR are obtained. The procedure involves making a small incision in the amniotic sac with an amnihook. Labor is shortened, and contractions increase in intensity. After the procedure, the mother and fetus are monitored closely along with assessing for complications.

Episiotomy: An episiotomy is a surgical incision of the perineum. This is performed to increase the size of the perineal outlet during birth. After the procedure, apply ice and assess the incision site. Teach the patient the importance of perineal care. Pain medications and Sitz baths are used to decrease discomfort. Complications such as infection and blood loss can occur.

Forceps: Forceps are instruments that are used to assist the fetal head to deliver. Complications that can occur are caput succedaneum, cephalohematoma, facial lacerations, and cerebral edema. After the birth, assess the infant for any complications.

Vacuum Extraction: Suction is applied to the fetal head to assist extraction. The FHR is monitored throughout. The mother is advised to push while the suction is attached. Once the fetus is delivered, assess for complications.

Cesarean Birth: This is a surgical procedure in which an abdominal and uterine incision is made to deliver the fetus. Preoperatively, consents are signed, a Foley catheter is inserted, an epidural is administered, an IV site is started, and support is provided as the main nursing interventions. Postoperatively assess vital signs, inspect the incision site, palpate the fundus, administer the proper medications, encourage hydration, ambulate the patient, and assess for complications.

Complications of Labor and Delivery

Preterm Labor

Definition: This is labor before the 37th week of gestation. Preterm labor can be caused by infection, drug or alcohol abuse, adolescent pregnancy, or complications.

Signs and Symptoms: Contractions, ruptured membranes, pelvic pressure, vaginal bleeding, and engagement of the fetus before the 37th week of gestation.

Diagnostics: Monitoring of uterine contractions.

Drug Therapy: Tocolytics are administered in an attempt to stop uterine contractions. Betamethasone is used to stimulate fetal lung development. IV fluids are used to hydrate the patient.

Nursing Care: Continue to monitor uterine contractions and the FHR. Administer medications as ordered. Monitor intake and output. The patient is maintained on bed rest, and hydration is encouraged. Monitor for complications, and report to physician if needed.

Abruptio Placenta

Definition: The placenta separates from the uterus before delivery. Abruptio placenta is caused by trauma, infection, drug use, and hypertension.

Signs and Symptoms: Dark red blood, uterus is firm, abdominal pain, and fetal distress can occur.

Diagnostics: Labs such as PT/PTT are done to assess clotting factors.

Complications: Hemorrhage, DIC, renal failure, shock, maternal and fetal death.

Drug Therapy: Blood transfusions are needed to treat blood loss.

Nursing Care: Monitor vital signs and blood loss, administer blood if needed, assess FHR, and prepare the patient for an emergency cesarean if a significant portion of the placenta has torn away from the uterine wall. Administer oxygen and IV fluids preoperatively. Monitor for complications.

Placenta Previa

Definition: The placenta is implanted in the lower uterine wall where it partially or completely covers the internal os of the cervix.

Signs and Symptoms: Blood is bright red, painless, abdomen is soft, and FHR may be within normal limits.

Diagnostics: Ultrasound is used for diagnosis.

Complications: Hemorrhage, shock, anemia, and fetal distress.

Drug Therapy: Blood products, betamethasone, and IV fluids.

Nursing Care: Monitor vital signs and blood loss; administer blood if needed; administer IVF; monitor FHR, intake, and output. Vaginal exams are contraindicated with this disorder. Continue to monitor bleeding, and report any complications to the primary care provider.

Prolapsed Umbilical Cord

Definition: The umbilical cord is prolapsed between the presenting part and the cervix. Immediate delivery is necessary due to the increased risks to the newborn.

Signs and Symptoms: FHR changes, fetal hypoxia, and the umbilical cord may present through the vaginal opening.

Diagnostics: Fetal monitoring and palpation of the umbilical cord.

Complications: Decreased fetal circulation, hypoxia, and fetal death.

Nursing Care: Prepare the mother for surgery. Relieve cord pressure while continuing to monitor the FHR. Oxygen is administered to the mother to treat fetal hypoxia. The mother may be placed in the Trendelenburg position to relieve pressure, or an examiner may hold the fetal head off the cord vaginally.

Precipitous Labor

Definition: Precipitous labor occurs when delivery of the infant is completed in less than 3 hours due to rapid dilation.

Signs and Symptoms: Frequent contractions with rapid descent of fetus.

Diagnostics: Continuous fetal monitoring.

Complications: Hemorrhage, vaginal laceration, hypoxia, and fetal trauma.

Drug Therapy: Tocolytic medications are administered.

Nursing Care: Preparation for delivery is done immediately. Supplies for delivery are prepared at the bedside. Continue to monitor the FHR. Stay with the mother at all times. Administer oxygen and tocolytics as ordered. Provide emotional support to the mother.

Shoulder Dystocia

Definition: This refers to prevention of delivery because the fetal shoulder being wedged under the maternal pubic bone.

Signs and Symptoms: During labor, the infant's head presents, but is retracted because passage of the shoulders is obstructed.

Diagnostics: Fetus unable to be delivered vaginally.

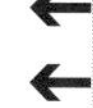

Complications: **Fracture of the clavicle or humerus.**

Nursing Care: Call an emergency. **Use McRoberts maneuvers by pulling the mother's knees toward her ears and flexing the thighs.** Use suprapubic pressure to fold the fetal shoulder toward the fetal chest. This maneuver can facilitate delivery by relieving pressure on the shoulders. An episiotomy may be performed to increase the vaginal opening to facilitate delivery. Prepare the mother and family for surgery if necessary. Continue to monitor the FHR assessing for complications.

Intrauterine Fetal Death

Definition: This refers to the death of the fetus while in utero due to a variety of complications that occur during the intrapartum stages.

Signs and Symptoms: Absence of fetal heart and movement.

Diagnostic: Ultrasound.

Complications: DIC can occur.

Drug Therapy: A platelet transfusion may be needed if DIC occurs.

Nursing Care: Prepare to deliver the fetus. Provide support for both the mother and the family. Assess and provide for the family's wishes. Monitor for complications and transfuse if necessary. Most hospitals have memory boxes that are often offered to the family. You will be able to see a memory box during clinical. These memory boxes are filled with keepsakes such as a lock of hair, photos, a blanket, and a crib card.

THE POSTPARTUM EXPERIENCE

Assessment of the Postpartum Woman

Uterus

Involution occurs during the postpartum stage, in which the uterus rapidly returns to its normal size. Assessment of the uterus is done every 8 hours, but more often initially. The fundus should be firm and under the umbilicus immediately after birth. If boggy, this can signify that the uterus is not contracting or involuting back down to its original position. Breastfeeding stimulates oxytocin, which increases involution. The fundus can also be massaged until firm.

Lochia

The uterus expels blood and debris after birth. The discharge changes in color as the uterus returns to the normal state, and documentation of the lochia is needed. From the day of delivery to the third day postpartum, a red discharge is seen, which is termed lochia rubra. For 4 to 10 days postpartum, the discharge is a brownish pink and is termed lochia serosa. During days 10 to 14, a white discharge is seen, which is called lochia alba. To assess lochia, a perineal pad is placed in the patient's underwear. Note the color and amount for documentation.

Nursing Care for Postpartum Women

Care of Afterbirth Pains

Afterbirth pains are contractions that occur after delivery due to involution. Women who breastfeed may have increased afterbirth pains. Ibuprofen is the drug of choice to treat pain.

Care of Perineal Discomfort

The perineal area may look edematous and reddened after delivery. Ice packs are applied to decrease swelling and discomfort. Sitz baths are advised to relieve discomfort, usually after the first 24 hours. Teach the patient to decrease infection by using a perineal bottle to clean the area after using the bathroom.

Care of Hemorrhoids

Administer stool softeners if needed. Advise the patient to increase fiber and fluid intake.

Care of Breastfeeding Discomfort

Treat breast soreness with warm showers, analgesics, and ice. Advise the patient to wear a supportive bra.

Assessment of Homan's Sign

Thrombophlebitis is a complication that can occur after delivery due to the hypercoagulability state of pregnancy. Manifestations are pain during dorsiflexion of the foot or pain during stretching of the legs. This is assessed every shift. An ultrasound is done to confirm diagnosis.

Postpartum Complications

Hemorrhage

Definition: Postpartum hemorrhage occurs after the delivery of the newborn, and is blood loss of 500 mL or more. It can result from hematoma, lacerations, uterine atony, or retained placenta.

Signs and Symptoms: Loss of substantial blood, fatigue, weakness, decreased blood levels, abdominal pain, and hypovolemia.

Diagnostics: Hematocrit and hemoglobin levels reveal blood loss.

Complications: Loss of consciousness and death.

Drug Therapy: Oxytocin (Pitocin) is administered along with blood products. Carboprost tromethamine (Hemabate) is used to treat postpartum hemorrhage.

Nursing Care: Monitor blood loss. Assess for shock or any changes in consciousness. **Treat uterine bogginess by massaging until firm**. Assess the fundus frequently. Administer medications as ordered. Obtain consent for blood products. Continue to monitor patient and labs.

Thrombophlebitis

Definition: Formation of a blood clot that causes inflammation on the venous wall. Deep vein thrombosis can occur after delivery.

Signs and Symptoms: **Lower extremity is swollen; tenderness and pain occur when the foot is dorsiflexed (positive Homan's sign); decreased pulse, and fever.**

Diagnostics: Doppler ultrasound is used to assess for thrombophlebitis.

Complications: Pulmonary embolism is a complication.

Drug Therapy: IV heparin or enoxaparin (Lovenox) and analgesics are administered.

Nursing Care: The patient is placed immediately on bed rest. Administer medications as ordered. Monitor labs such as PT/INR when the patient is placed on heparin or Lovenox. Monitor the patient closely when placed on an IV heparin drip, maintaining bleeding precautions. The affected leg is elevated. **Teach the patient not to massage the site, cross legs, or apply pressure**. Monitor for complications, and teach the patient ways to prevent further blood clots.

Postpartum Infections

Definition: Women are at increased risk for infection during the postpartum stage. Infections such as UTI and infections of the perineal or cesarean incision are common.

Signs and Symptoms: Fever, pain at the site, foul-smelling lochia, chills, weight loss, pain, and drainage.

Diagnostics: White blood cell (WBC) and wound cultures can diagnose an infection.

Complications: If left untreated, infection can become systemic.

Drug Therapy: Antibiotics, analgesics, and pain management.

Nursing Care: Monitor labs and administer medications as ordered. Monitor vital signs every 4 hours or more often if needed. Administer IV fluids, and encourage the patient to increase fluid intake. Assess the incision, and change dressing as ordered.

Mastitis

Definition: Mastitis is infection of the connective tissue in the breast that occurs in lactating women. **Candida albicans is the causative organism.** ←

Signs and Symptoms: Fever and headache; breast is sore and painful.

Diagnostics: Culture of the breast milk and clinical symptoms.

Complications: Breast abscess can occur if left untreated.

Drug Therapy: Antibiotics, analgesics, and pain management.

Nursing Care: Assess breasts for pain and redness. Apply heat and advise the patient to wear a supportive bra. Administer medications as ordered.

Postpartum Depression

Definition: Depression that occurs during the postpartum stage.

Signs and Symptoms: Crying, loss of interest, loss of appetite, insomnia, racing thoughts, suicidal ideation, and lack of concentration.

Diagnostics: Clinical symptoms and postpartum depression scale.

Complications: Suicide can occur if depression worsens.

Drug Therapy: Antidepressants.

Nursing Care: If symptoms do not resolve on their own, the patient may be referred to a mental health professional. Treatment options will then be discussed—either therapy or medication. The nursing responsibilities are to monitor for these symptoms, follow up with the patient, and refer the patient to the correct facility for further treatment. Family teaching is necessary.

THE NEWBORN ASSESSMENT

The Newborn's Physical Exam

After delivery, suction the infant and place on a warming table. An Apgar score is done at 1 minute and then at 5 minutes. Vital signs are obtained frequently immediately after birth, usually every 15 minutes. Normal findings are pulse of 110 to 150, respirations of 30 to 60, and temperature of 97.6 °F.

Skin

The skin should appear pink, soft, and warm, with lanugo covering the back and face. Assess for Mongolian spots, acrocyanosis, milia, and jaundice.

Head

The size, shape, and symmetry are noted. The head is measured in relation to the chest. The fontanels are palpated. Molding, caput succedaneum, and cephalhematoma are documented, if present.

Eyes, Ears, and Nose

Assess symmetry of the eyes. Assess pupils for color, reaction to light, and movements of lids. Assess for drainage, subconjunctival hemorrhage, retinal hemorrhage, strabismus, and conjunctivitis. The eyelids may appear edematous due to the pressure from delivery. An erythromycin ointment is applied to the eyes to protect against *Neisseria gonorrhea* and *Chlamydia*. Assess the ears for symmetry. Low-set ears are sometimes a sign of congenital anomalies. Inspect the nose for shape, size, and symmetry. The nose should be midline and patent.

Mouth and Neck

Assess the mouth for signs of cleft lip or palate. Look for symmetry of the lips. Assess the palate for the presence of Epstein "pearls" (tiny white lesions) that may be seen on the hard palate. Assess the mouth for signs of thrush, a white substance found on the tongue. Ensure the uvula is intact and midline. Assess the infant's swallowing and sucking reflex. The neck should appear short; the infant does not have the ability to support his or her head. Palpate the neck for any lesions. The clavicles should be assessed for fractures that could be caused by delivery. Document any findings.

Chest

An overall assessment of the chest is done. The thorax should be symmetrical. Assess for any signs of respiratory difficulties such as retractions or labored breathing. Auscultations of breath sounds are performed. Assess and palpate the breast tissue while assessing the nipples. Secretions from the nipples are normal at this time.

Abdomen and Umbilical Cord

The shape of the abdomen appears protuberant and moves with each respiration. Assess for abdominal distension or abnormalities that may be present. Auscultation of bowel sounds is performed; bowel sounds are commonly heard immediately after birth.

The umbilical cord appears white. Two umbilical arteries and one umbilical vein are normal. Assess for signs of umbilical hernia, and contact the primary care provider if present. Provide cord care based on policy.

Genitals

In girls, assess the labia majora, labia minora, and clitoris. Vaginal bleeding and discharge may be seen in infants due to the maternal hormones in the infant system. In males, assess the overall appearance of the penis. The penis should have a foreskin covering its tip, the scrotum may appear edematous, and the testes should be descended. Assess for complications such as inguinal hernia, cryptorchidism, and hydrocele. Assess the anal area and ascertain whether the opening is visually patent. Document the first meconium stool that occurs during the first 24 hours of birth.

Extremities and Spine

Assess both lower and upper extremities. Assess the hands and feet by counting the digits, confirming 10 toes and 10 fingers. Perform range of motion on the arms and hands, assessing for any complications. Inspect the hands for the presence of palmar creases. Palpate brachial pulses. Assess the lower extremities for symmetry. Assess for hip dislocation using the Ortolani and Barlow maneuvers. Ensure the gluteal folds are symmetrical. Assess the feet for any deformities such as talipes equinovarus (foot turns inward and downward). Assess for sole creases, and document the findings. Assess the spine for symmetry and complications.

Review of Systems

Respiratory System

The normal respiratory rate is 30 to 60. Assess the infant's breathing pattern, noting any changes or difficulty. Auscultate breath sounds, assessing for any crackles or wheezing. Suction the infant if necessary. Check the peripheral pulse oximetry.

Cardiovascular System

The normal pulse ranges from 110 to 150 bpm. Palpate the apical pulse. Auscultate for any murmurs or thrills. Acrocyanosis (blue hands/feet) is normal for 24 hours after birth.

Gastrointestinal System

Assess for meconium stool. The newborn's stomach is very small and does not require large amounts of formula or breast milk. As the infant grows, the demand for more food will occur.

Assess for sucking, rooting, and swallowing reflexes before feedings. Difficulty with feedings should be documented and reported to the physician for further assessment.

Genitourinary System

Monitor the newborn's intake and output. This may be done by weighing the diaper. Weigh the infant daily. Monitor for complications such as dehydration.

Neurological System

Assess head circumference and palpate fontanels. Perform all newborn reflexes while assessing muscle tone. The palmar and plantar grasp are usually evaluated by placing a finger in the palm of the hand or toes; the fingers/toes should curl around the finger. The Babinski sign tests the plantar reflex by gently stroking the foot; in response extension of the toes occurs. The sucking, rooting, and swallowing reflexes are evaluated by gently touching the side of the cheek of the newborn to elicit the rooting reflex, then placing a finger in the newborn's mouth to elicit the sucking reflex, and ensuring that the infant can swallow either breast milk or formula without any difficulty. The Moro reflex is elicited by startling the infant to elicit a response. The infant will then extend the arms, flex hands, and return to its relaxed state.

Newborn Complications

Premature Newborn

Definition: Infant born before 37 weeks of gestation.

→ *Signs and Symptoms:* **Respiratory difficulty, hypothermia, hypoxia, absent reflexes, jaundice, skin thin, bowel sounds are absent or diminished, poor feeding, decrease in urine output, low birth weight, and testes do not descend in males.**

Diagnostics: Physical assessment can determine gestational age.

Complications: Respiratory difficulty, hypoxemia, hypoglycemia, aspiration, and infection.

Nursing Care: Monitor vital signs frequently. Administer oxygen if needed, while continuously monitoring the respirations. Place infant under warmer. Perform feedings on a scheduled basis. Monitor intake and output. If severe dehydration is present, IV fluids may be administered. Obtain a blood glucose level. Prevent infection due to the infant's increased risk. Teach the parents that skin-to-skin interaction is important at this time.

Small for Gestational Age (SGA)

Definition: Newborns who are born on the lower spectrum of the birth weight are termed SGA. Low birth weights can be caused by intrauterine growth restriction (IUGR), maternal high blood pressure, maternal smoking or alcohol usage during pregnancy, and heart disease.

Signs and Symptoms: Hypoglycemia, cyanosis, small physical appearance, difficulty feeding, and infant may appear jaundiced.

Diagnostics: Blood glucose levels and physical assessment.

Complications: Hypothermia, hypoglycemia, polycythemia, aspiration syndrome, cyanosis, and infection.

Nursing Care: Monitor for complications directly after birth. Administer oxygen if needed. Place the infant under the warmer to prevent hypothermia. Obtain a blood glucose level; if results are low, administer feedings/glucose either orally or intravenously. Provide feedings on a scheduled basis. Continue to monitor vital signs, weight, intake, and output. Continue to monitor for complications.

Large for Gestational Age (LGA)

Definition: This refers to newborns who are born above the 90th percentile of birth weight. A LGA infant can be caused by maternal glucose instability or multiparous women.

Signs and Symptoms: Hypoglycemia, physical appearance, trauma from birth, and poor feeding.

Diagnostics: Weight and physical appearance can diagnose LGA.

Complications: Fractured clavicles, hypoglycemia, polycythemia, and infection.

Nursing Care: Monitor vital signs. Assess for complications after birth such as clavicle fractures or trauma from birth. Obtain a blood glucose level, and treat as ordered. Begin regular scheduled feedings. Continue to monitor infant for complications.

Respiratory Distress Syndrome (RDS)

Definition: This severe respiratory disorder is caused by a decrease in surfactant in preterm infants.

Signs and Symptoms: Tachypnea, retractions, nasal flaring, decreased breath sounds, apnea, cyanosis, hypothermia, grunting, and hypoxemia.

Diagnostics: Chest x-ray can diagnose RDS.

Complications: Respiratory acidosis, severe hypoxia, and respiratory failure can occur.

Drug Therapy: Administration of oxygen and surfactant is used.

Nursing Care:

Monitor respirations, vital signs, and O_2 saturations. Administer oxygen as ordered. Ventilation may be needed in severe cases. Obtain arterial blood gases.

Initiate feedings with periods of rest to conserve energy. The infant should be positioned on his or her side to facilitate better breathing. Family teaching is necessary.

Meconium Aspiration Syndrome

Definition: Meconium aspiration occurs when meconium is released into the amniotic fluid, causing the infant to aspirate during birth.

Signs and Symptoms: Hypoxia, cyanosis, nasal flaring, crackles, tachypnea, decreased pulse, diminished breath sounds, barrel chest, and stained skin.

Diagnostics: Chest x-ray and arterial blood gases.

Complications: Respiratory failure, infection, pneumothorax, and hypoxia.

Drug Therapy: IV fluids and oxygen are administered.

Nursing Care: Once the infant is born, immediate suctioning is performed. The infant's respiratory status is closely monitored. Continue to maintain a patent airway. If the infant is suffering from severe meconium aspiration syndrome, he or she is placed in the NICU with continuous monitoring. Ventilation may be needed to maintain an open airway.

Jaundice

→ *Definition:* **Jaundice is caused by an increase in unconjugated bilirubin**. Jaundice is commonly seen in the first 24 hours of life.

Signs and Symptoms: Yellow tint to the skin and sclera, dehydration, poor feeding, fatigue, and frequent stools.

Diagnostics: Serum bilirubin levels, urinalysis, Coombs' test, CBC, and testing of Rh or ABO incompatibility is used to confirm diagnosis.

Complications: Kernicterus, hearing loss, anemia, and developmental delays.

Drug Therapy: IV fluids are administered to treat dehydration.

Nursing Care: If jaundice is present, contact the physician and do a complete assessment of the infant. Phototherapy is the first line of treatment. **Phototherapy involves placing the infant under a set of fluorescent lights to decrease bilirubin levels.** During phototherapy, the infant's eyes and genitals are covered. Monitor the infant's hydration, skin, and vital signs. Continue to monitor labs and serum bilirubin levels. Maintain feedings and monitor bowel movements.

Hypoglycemia

Definition: Normal blood glucose levels are 50 to 80 mg/dL. Hypoglycemia is diagnosed when the infant's blood glucose level is lower than 30 to 45 mg/dL.

Signs and Symptoms: Poor feeding, high-pitched cry, tremors, a decrease in temperature, and irregular respirations.

Diagnostics: Blood glucose levels.

Complications: Seizures, respiratory distress, hypocalcemia, and hypothermia.

Drug Therapy: IV glucose or D5W can be administered intravenously.

Nursing Care: Monitor blood glucose levels. Oral feedings are administered before IV glucose. Maintain a patient airway. Monitor for complications.

Fetal Alcohol Syndrome (FAS)

Definition: Fetal alcohol syndrome occurs in infants as a result of maternal alcohol abuse during pregnancy. FAS is the leading cause of mental retardation.

Signs and Symptoms: **Tremors, hypoglycemia, respiratory distress, irritability, broad nasal bridge, abdominal distension, difficulty feeding, and abnormal reflexes.**

Diagnostics: Presentation of symptoms and maternal alcohol history.

Complications: Seizures, mental retardation, failure to thrive, low IQ, and cognitive impairment.

Nursing Care: Ensure a patent airway. Maintain seizure precautions. Monitor vital signs. Monitor for complications. Infants usually go through withdrawal within 3 days of birth. Suction secretions if needed. The infant should be swaddled tightly while in the nursery. Feeding should be scheduled, with frequent burping.

Neonatal Abstinence Syndrome (NAS)

Definition: Neonatal abstinence syndrome occurs in infants born to mothers who used or abused drugs during pregnancy. The drugs are passed on to the infant through the placenta.

Signs and Symptoms: Tremors, high-pitched cry, respiratory distress, sneezing, poor feeding, low birth weight, increased muscle tone, vomiting, diarrhea, and fever.

Diagnostics: Maternal drug history and clinical symptoms.

Complications: Respiratory distress, seizures, low birth weight, infection, and developmental delays.

Drug Therapy: IVF is administered to maintain hydration.

Nursing Care: Maintain seizure precautions. Keep the room quiet and decrease stimuli. Swaddle the infant. Regular scheduled feedings are administered. Administer IVF as ordered. Monitor vital signs routinely. The infant will begin withdrawal soon after birth. Assess the infant for complications that could arise.

Newborns With HIV/AIDS

Definition: Infants can contract HIV/AIDS through the maternal blood supply.

Signs and Symptoms: The infants can be asymptomatic for a long time. If symptoms are present, an enlarged spleen, liver, and glands are seen. Other symptoms include GI upset, respiratory infection, and growth delays.

Diagnostics: Ultrasound, ELISA test, and western blot test are used for the HIV/AIDS–infected mother and newborns.

Complications: Respiratory infections and failure to thrive.

Drug Therapy: Antiretroviral medication is administered right after birth. A CBC is done to confirm that HIV was not transmitted.

Nursing Care: Caring for the mother and newborn is not much different. Handwashing is important to decrease the risk of infection. The infants are given vitamin K, antiretrovirals, and immunizations. The mother continues her medication as prescribed. Do not administer live vaccines to HIV-infected newborns. Breastfeeding is not recommended. Feedings are administered on a scheduled basis. Monitor for complications. Frequent visits to the doctor are needed for the first few months after birth. Family teaching is needed before discharge.

MATERNITY PHARMACOLOGY

AquaMEPHYTON (Vitamin K)

Definition: This is used to prevent hemorrhage in newborns due to insufficient prothrombin levels.

Side Effects: Pain at the injection site, swelling, and bleeding.

Nursing Care: Vitamin K is administered in the vastus lateralis thigh muscle. Monitor for side effects and complications such as bleeding. The medication is light sensitive and should be kept in a brown glass vial.

Betamethasone

Definition: This is administered to increase respiratory development in newborns who lack surfactant.

Side Effects: Infection, increase in blood glucose, and edema are common side effects.

Nursing Care: Betamethasone is administered through IM injections. Assess the site for pain or swelling. Continue to monitor the fetus. Monitor for side effects and complications.

Erythromycin Ointment

Definition: This is a prophylactic eye ointment that is used to decrease the risk of neonatal conjunctivitis from *Neisseria gonorrhea* and *Chlamydia*.

Side Effects: Blindness.

Nursing Care: Erythromycin is administered shortly after birth. Wash hands and clean the newborn's eyes before administration. Apply the ointment to the lower lid. Assess for side effects or reaction to the medication.

Magnesium Sulfate

Definition: This is used to decrease preeclampsia by relaxing smooth muscle. Magnesium sulfate is also used to slow contractions during preterm labor.

Side Effects: GI upset, headache, respiratory depression, sweating, hypotension, and decreased reflexes.

Nursing Care: Magnesium sulfate is administered through IV infusion. Frequent checks of vital signs and close monitoring of the fetus are important during administration. Monitor for complications such as cardiac arrest and respiratory depression that can occur with magnesium toxicity. Monitor urine output, and report if less than 30 mL of urine during an hour. Assess deep tendon reflexes.

Oxytocin (Pitocin)

Definition: Oxytocin (Pitocin) is used to stimulate labor and increase uterine contractions. It is used for postpartum hemorrhage.

Side Effects: Hemorrhage, water intoxication, hypotension, rapid labor, and cardiac arrhythmias.

Nursing Care: Oxytocin is administered through IV infusion. Monitor maternal vital signs, uterine contractions, and fetal heart tones during administration. Document and assess IV rate as prescribed. Monitor for complications, and report symptoms to the primary care provider.

Pain Management

Types: Butorphanol (Stadol) and nalbuphine hydrochloride (Nubain)

Definition: Narcotics are used to control pain during labor. Can be administered IV or IM. The antidote for narcotics is naloxone (Narcan).

Side Effects: GI upset, drowsiness, hypotension, urinary retention, respiratory depression, and vision disturbances.

Nursing Care: Monitor vital signs and fetal heart tones before administration. Monitor urine output. Monitor for side effects and complications. Narcan should be available for emergency use.

Prostaglandins

Types: Dinoprostone (Cervidil and Prepidil).

Definition: They are used to stimulate labor and increase uterine contractions. Prostaglandins are administered vaginally.

Side Effects: GI upset, headache, hypotension, rapid labor, and fever.

Nursing Care: Monitor maternal vital signs, contractions, and → fetal heart tones. **Administer medication vaginally, and have the patient lie on her side for 30 minutes.** Prepare the mother and family for delivery. Administer medications for pain as prescribed. Monitor for side effects and complications.

Rho (D) Immune Globulin (RhoGAM)

Definition: RhoGAM is administered to Rh-negative patients who may have been exposed to the Rh-positive antibody. RhoGAM is given intramuscularly.

Side Effects: Swelling and pain at the injection site. Do not administer medication to Rh-positive women.

Nursing Care: If the patient has been exposed to Rh-positive blood, then RhoGAM is administered twice during pregnancy. If the infant is exposed to Rh positive, RhoGAM is administered within 72 hours.

EIGHT

PSYCHIATRIC NURSING

Psychiatric nursing involves working with individuals with various mental disorders. I am sure you have experienced anxiety at one time or another. Can you imagine experiencing anxious feelings all day? Can you imagine feeling sad all day? These are real emotions and disorders that many people suffer with. Much stigma is attached to mental illnesses and to individuals who suffer from them, and many misconceptions prevail about them. These false beliefs and fears may also be present in student nurses. However, as you become acquainted with psychiatric patients and begin to understand the basics of mental illness, this stigma will decrease.

In psychiatric nursing, you will continue to use the med–surg skills when necessary, but the real focus is upon therapeutic use of self. You will learn how to use words, body language, and the milieu to facilitate healing for patients with mental illness. Psychopharmacology, electroconvulsive therapy (ECT), light therapy, vagal nerve stimulation, and transmagnetic stimulation of the brain are some procedures used to treat psychiatric disorders. Individuals experiencing mental illness are encountered not only in psychiatric facilities, but also in any area where you practice, as well as in your community. The skills you develop in psychiatric nursing will be transferable to any setting. You will learn the basics of supportive therapy using therapeutic communication, assessment of common signs and symptoms of mental illness, and multiple treatment modalities that you have not previously seen. It is important to establish a therapeutic nurse–client relationship to understand and correctly treat these disorders.

The course will expose you to the various disorders that exist in psychiatric nursing. These patients may exhibit both physical and emotional symptoms. Although no medical problems may be assessed on initial examination, a patient's symptoms may be exacerbated by the severe mental stressors. Most of the time, patients are tested extensively for a cause of these symptoms, but usually a medical cause cannot be determined. An example is the patient who comes into the ER with a severe panic disorder and spends several hours in the ER before learning that no medical cause has been identified. Discouraged, these patients often return home to deal with these symptoms on their own unless properly referred to a mental health facility or practitioner.

The exams in the course are similar to the other courses in which the content is based on various disorders, symptoms, and treatments. The first exam is commonly based on your knowledge of maintaining a therapeutic relationship with psychiatric patients. This section of the course is very important; it will teach you the ability to communicate on a therapeutic level.

The clinical portion of this course is very different from the other clinical experiences. Patients are usually ambulatory and are involved in group as well as individual therapy, and participate in various recreational and artistic activities to facilitate coping with their symptoms. Families usually are usually involved, as well, and psychoeducation is very important.

Schizophrenia

Definition: A series of disorders characterized by a thought disorder resulting in perceptual distortions or a break from reality. Approximately 1% of the population has the genetic predisposition (dopamine abnormality) for schizophrenia, and when this predisposition is combined with stressors, symptoms often develop. Because of perceptual distortions associated with the disorder, patients often have difficulty functioning or meeting basic needs and may demonstrate erratic/agitated behavior. These symptoms also result in social skill deficits and often depression and anxiety.

Signs and Symptoms: Hallucinations, delusions, flat affect, algolia (diminished thoughts), lack of motivation, impaired judgment, inability to make decisions, withdrawn, erratic behavior, paranoia, poor hygiene, loss of appetite, poor sleeping habits, difficulty with speech, and suicidal thoughts.

Diagnostics: Clinical examination based on the *DSM-5* diagnostic criteria.

Complications: A decrease in quality of life, suicidal thoughts, and danger to self and others.

Drug Therapy: Antipsychotics, antiepileptic, antianxiety, and antidepressants are used.

Nursing Interventions: Safety is first and most important. Avoid large groups and overstimulation. Avoid encouraging delusional ideas, and bring the patient back to a state of reality.

If the patient is experiencing suicidal thoughts, precautions are needed along with frequent monitoring. ECT can also be used to treat symptoms, especially if catatonic. Administer medications as ordered while assessing for side effects. Owing to long-term treatment, side effects are common. Poor compliance is often a problem. Social rehabilitation is important when the disorder is chronic. Cognitive behavioral therapy is used to cope with the symptoms, as well as supportive therapy for patients and families.

Generalized Anxiety Disorder (GAD)

Definition: A group of disorders characterized by state of worry that occurs over a long period of time. The symptoms contribute to a decrease of participation in activities of daily life, owing to the constant state of worry. Anxiety can vary from mild to a state of panic with intensifying symptoms at each stage. Obsessive-compulsive disorder adds repetitive thoughts (e.g., preoccupied with germs or locking doors) and actions (e.g., repeatedly washing hands, rechecking doors multiple times) to the anxiety and is a long-term disorder.

Signs and Symptoms: Trembling, increased heart rate, cold hands/feet, sweating, palpitations, dizziness, impending doom, irritability, fatigue, frequent urination, impaired concentration, shortness of breath, chest pain, vision changes, decreased attention span, muscle tension, and GI upset.

Diagnostics: Based on clinical examination and *DSM* categories. GAD is diagnosed if the patient's symptoms persist for more than 6 months.

Complications: Panic disorder, suicidal thoughts, and depression can occur if symptoms persist.

Drug Therapy: Benzodiazepines and selective serotonin reuptake inhibitors (SSRIs) are commonly used to treat GAD.

Nursing Interventions: If the patient is experiencing an anxious episode, stay with the patient and use breathing techniques to calm the patient. Decrease stimuli. Administer medication as ordered. Refer patient for cognitive therapy if needed.

Depression

Definition: A group of clinical disorders characterized primarily by an abnormal mood; can develop at any age from childhood to old age. Mood is a pervasive feeling that is experienced subjectively and influences thoughts, behaviors, physical sensations, and perceptions. A depressed mood is different from brief passing sadness or grief after a loss. A decrease in the necessary levels of serotonin in the CNS combined with environmental stressors is believed to be the cause.

Signs and Symptoms: Usual symptoms include changes in mood as well as vegetative symptoms. Mood changes include sadness, despair, sense of emptiness, anhedonia (loss of ability to enjoy pleasure), low self-esteem, excessive emotional sensitivity, pessimistic thinking, irritability, excessive guilt, indecisiveness, and often suicidal thoughts. Vegetative symptoms includes disturbance of sleep (difficulty falling asleep, middle of the night or early morning awakening), increase or decrease in appetite with weight gain or loss, lack of motivation and difficulty functioning in all aspects of life. There is a dramatic change in usual mood.

Diagnostics: Clinical examination using *DSM*. There are many self-reports as well as structured interviews to assist with diagnosis.

Complications: Suicide, increased physical problems, especially in the elderly, and slower healing from surgery.

Drug Therapy: Antidepressants (SSRIs used first), antianxiety, and sleep medications. If unresponsive, an antipsychotic may be added to the antidepressant.

Nursing Interventions: Provide safety. Develop a crisis plan if suicidal thoughts increase. Encourage involvement in therapy as well as medications. Cognitive behavioral therapy to reduce depressive thoughts has been successful in decreasing recurrences and as a problem-solving approach and supportive therapy. Exercise and well-balanced meals are also important in preventing recurrences. Use of a full spectrum light box is effective for seasonal affective disorder. Psychoeducation with family is important. Encourage involvement in self-help groups.

Bipolar Disorder

Definition: A disorder that varies from manic to depressive episodes. If the depressive and manic episodes are very mild, it is labeled cyclothymic.

Signs and Symptoms: Mania may be characterized by euphoria or irritability, grandiosity or increased self-esteem, decreased need for sleep, racing thoughts with pressured speech, increased activity, poor judgment involving spending sprees, promiscuity, gambling, or other unusual behaviors. Mania symptoms may range from mild hypomania to full-blown mania. Depressive symptoms are the same as in depressive illness.

Diagnostics: Based on symptoms of mania and depressive episodes. Various depression scales may be used to make a diagnosis.

Complications: Erratic behavior can be harmful to the patient or others. The patient may experience suicidal thoughts.

Drug Therapy: Mood stabilizers such as lithium, SSRIs, and benzodiazepines are often prescribed. Antidepressants should always be ordered with a mood stabilizer to avoid activation of mania. Poor compliance is often an issue.

Nursing Interventions: Monitor the patient frequently and closely owing to rapid changes in mood. Keep the patient and others away from harmful objects or situations. Administer medications as prescribed, assessing for side effects. Encourage the patient to maintain a regular diet with periods of rest. During periods of erratic behavior, stay with the patient and decrease stimuli. Assistance may be needed if the patient's behavior becomes combative or violent.

Personality Disorder

Definition: A disruption within personality traits that leads to functional impairment and behavioral instability. There are several types of personality disorders that are organized by clusters.

Types: Cluster A consists of odd behaviors such as paranoid, schizoid, and schizotypal personality disorders. Cluster B is described as emotional or erratic behavior, such as antisocial, borderline, histrionic, and narcissistic personality disorders. Cluster C are anxious or scared behaviors termed avoidant, dependent, or obsessive-compulsive personality disorder. The patient's symptoms are used to diagnose the type of cluster for the particular personality disorder.

Cluster A Clinical Signs: Delusions, withdrawn behavior, hallucinations, magical thinking, flat affect, disorganized speech, suspiciousness, combativeness, and paranoia. ←

Cluster B Clinical Signs: Self-centered attitude, inappropriate attire, dramatic change in behavior, anxiety, depression, withdrawal, easily distracted, and manipulative. ←

→ **Cluster C Clinical Signs: Anxious, withdrawn, ritualistic, impulsive, irritable, and tends to lack social skills.**

Diagnostics: Personality disorders are diagnosed with reference to the *DSM-5* criteria.

Complications: Erratic behavior can lead to harm to self or others and low functioning.

Drug Therapy: SSRIs, monoamine oxidase inhibitors (MAOIs), and antipsychotics can be used to increase stability and functioning.

Nursing Interventions: Provide a safe environment for the patient with frequent monitoring to prevent self-destructive actions. Help the patient recognize erratic behavior and coach him or her through these behaviors. Encourage the patient to attend meetings or keep a journal to write down his or her feelings. Maintain trust and avoid behaviors that may make the patient hostile. Cognitive behavioral therapy is also used along with medication to treat personality disorders. Administer medications as prescribed and assess for side effects.

DISORDERS IN THE ELDERLY POPULATION

Delirium

Definition: A sudden change in cognition that occurs throughout the day for short periods. Before treatment occurs, a cause must be identified. The causes of delirium are usually medication reactions, substance abuse, and lack of sleep.

Signs and Symptoms: Acute change in cognition lasting only a short time. Other symptoms are confusion, decreased level of attention, agitation, fatigue, and visual hallucinations.

Diagnostics: Mental status exam, EKG, EEG, CBC, ABGs, urine culture, drug screen, MRI, and CT scan. The reason for the abundant diagnostics is that in order to treat delirium, an underlying cause may first be identified.

Complications: Owing to the rapid change in cognition, the patient may experience suicidal thoughts. Maintain safety and implement precautions against suicide.

Drug Therapy: Once the underlying cause is found, medication is given to treat it.

Nursing Interventions: Maintain safety precautions. Perform a series of diagnostics to find an underlying cause. Treat the underlying cause rapidly and extensively. Obtain a health history from a family member if available. Provide support to both the patient and the family. Provide a safe environment.

Dementia/Alzheimer's Disease

Definition: Impaired cognition that progresses over time. Dementia can be caused by an organic brain disease, age, genetics, depression, and head trauma. Alzheimer's disease is a type of dementia caused by cell damage and is irreversible.

Signs and Symptoms: Confusion, disorientation, poor judgment, inability to make decisions, personality changes, sleep disturbances, poor nutrition, aphasia, incontinence, and inability to perform activities of daily life.

Diagnostics: CBC, urine test, drug screen, CT scan, MRI, EKG, and a lumbar puncture may be done to examine the spinal fluid.

Drug Therapy: Treatments for decreasing the progression of dementia and Alzheimer's disease are donepezil (Aricept), tacrine (Cognex), and rivastigmine (Exelon). Treatments for depression are SSRIs, commonly fluoxetine (Prozac) and paroxetine (Paxil).

Nursing Interventions: Dementia is a progressive disease, and treating the underlying cause can decrease progression during the early stages. Assist with ADLs, and devise strategies to assist memory. Encourage continued activity, including physical, social, and mental types. Help patients and their families with referrals to support groups.

PSYCHIATRIC MEDICATIONS

Antipsychotics

Types: There are two types of antipsychotics: typical (affecting dopamine levels) and atypical (affecting dopamine/serotonin) medications. Typical antipsychotics are chlorpromazine (Thorazine), haloperidol (Haldol), fluphenazine (Proxilin), thiothixene hydrochloride (Navane), loxapine (Loxitane), trifluoperazine (Stelazine), molidone (Mobane), and perphenazine (Trilaton). Atypical antipsychotics are risperidone (Risperdal), quetiapine (Seroquel), clozapine (Clozaril), olanzapine (Zyprexa), aripiprazole (Abilify), lurasidone (Latuda), iloperidone (Fanapt), asenapine (Saphris), and ziprasidone (Zeldox).

Definition: Antipsychotics treat the symptoms of patients who suffer from schizophrenia. These medications are used to decrease hallucinations, delusions, and erratic or violent behavior.

Contraindications: Patients with a history of cardiac problems are advised to use antipsychotics with caution.

Pharmacokinetics: Antipsychotics are orally prescribed per physician dosage. Take medication with food to decrease GI upset. Long-acting injections are available for several antipsychotics and are useful for patients who do not take medications as ordered. Some are also available in injection form and used to decrease agitation if oral medications are not effective.

→ *Side Effects:* **Antipsychotics can cause extrapyramidal symptoms that can present as pseudoparkinsonism, akinesia (stiffness), akathisia, dystonia, and tardive dyskinesia disorders. Parkinsonism presents as tremors, shuffling gait, drooling, and rigidity. Akathisia occurs days after taking the medication and presents as restlessness or not being able to sit still. Dystonia is spastic, uncontrollable muscular movements.**

Tardive dyskinesia develops after long-term use and involves bizarre dystonic movements of mouth, lips, limbs, and the entire body. This is due to the excessive stimulation of dopamine.

Neuroleptic malignant syndrome is a complication that can occur with antipsychotics. This complication is fatal and should be treated immediately. Symptoms are severe fever, tachycardia, sweating, blood pressure changes, dyspnea, seizures, extrapyramidal symptoms, and change in mental status. Treatment needs to occur immediately, a physician needs to be called, vital signs are monitored, I/O monitored, the medication stopped, mental status assessed, and the ordered medications administered.

Nursing Care: Teach correct medication dosage and side effects. Advise the patient to monitor for any complications or severe side effects and to report them immediately. Monitor vital signs, output, and input. Advise the patient to avoid alcohol or CNS depressants while on these medications. Patients should wear protective clothing when outdoors to avoid excessive sun exposure. Antipsychotics should not be discontinued abruptly but gradually decreased.

Antianxiety Medications

Types: Benzodiazepines such as alprazolam (Xanax), lorazepam (Ativan), diazepam (Valium), clonazepam (Klonopin), chlordiazepoxide (Librium), paroxetine (Paxil), midazolam (Versed), and oxazepam (Serax), as well as buspirone (BuSpar), which has a distinct chemical makeup.

Definition: Antianxiety medications are used to decrease symptoms of anxiety. Benzodiazepines are able to decrease anxiety through CNS depression.

Contraindications: Patients taking other CNS depressants or antipsychotics should speak to a physician before taking benzodiazepines.

Pharmacokinetics: Given orally with food to decrease GI upset.

Side Effects: Dizziness, sedation, headache, GI upset, agranulocytosis, change in mental status, and difficulty sleeping.

Nursing Care: Teach patients the importance of taking the proper dosage. Overdosing is common and can cause serious complications; teaching the patient the proper usage of benzodiazepines can prevent these occurrences. Patients can also have withdrawal symptoms if the medications are discontinued abruptly, and should therefore gradually decrease dosage per physician order. Advise the patient to take the medication at night owing to the side effect of sedation, and to avoid alcohol. Continue to monitor the patient and side effects throughout treatment.

Antidepressants

Types: Selective serotonin reuptake inhibitors (SSRIs), serotonin-norepinephrine reuptake inhibitors (SNRIs), tricyclic antidepressants (TCAs), and monoamine oxidase inhibitors (MAOIs).

Selective Serotonin Reuptake Inhibitors (SSRIs) and Serotonin-Norepinephrine Reuptake Inhibitors (SNRIs)

Types: SSRIs are citalopram (Celexa), fluoxetine (Prozac), escitalopram (Lexapro), fluvoxamine (Luvox), paroxetine (Paxil), and sertraline (Zoloft). SNRIs are duloxetine (Cymbalta), venlafaxine (Effexor), and desvenlafaxine (Pristiq).

Definition: Inhibit reuptake of serotonin at the synapse, resulting in increased levels of serotonin, thereby causing an antidepressant reaction. SSRIs are given to patients who suffer from depression or anxiety. SNRIs also prevent reuptake of norepinephrine. SNRIs are usually ordered if the SSRI is not effective.

Contraindications: Patients taking MAOIs and antipsychotics should use caution when taking SSRIs. The patient should be instructed to check with a provider before taking SSRIs; there are many medication contraindications. SNRIs may raise blood pressure as well as cause urinary retention

Pharmacokinetics: Given orally with food to decrease GI upset.

Side Effects: SSRIs have the fewest side effects of all the antidepressants. Side effects include GI upset, headache, dizziness, CNS effects, fatigue, weight changes, appetite changes, photosensitivity, sexual dysfunction, and nervousness. SNRIs may also cause urinary retention, dry mouth, dry eyes, orthostatic hypotension, and insomnia.

Nursing Care: Advise patients to take medication as ordered. It takes 2 to 4 weeks to begin to notice changes in vegetative signs, and later the mood improves. Remember that antidepressants are not " happy pills " and that therapy must be used to facilitate recovery as well as prevent future episodes. Many patients feel hopeless and stop the medications when there is no improvement in a few days. It is important to point out improvements to patients and families as they occur.

Assess for side effects, and if severe, contact the physician. Give medication with food to decrease GI upset. There are many medication contraindications; advise patients to use caution while taking SSRIs and to take the medication at night in case of dizziness. Assess blood pressure, and watch for a decrease in blood pressure when changing positions. Liver and renal function tests are monitored while on long-term therapy. Depressed patients are still at risk for suicide, so continue to monitor them during treatment.

Tricyclic Antidepressants (TCAs)

Types: Amitriptyline (Elavil), trazadone (Desyrel), butriptyline (Evadyne), clomipramine (Anafranil), doxepin (Adapin or Sinequan), imipramine (Tofranil), imipraminoxide (Imiprex), maprotiline (Ludiomil), trimipramine (Surmontil), desipramine (Norpramin), nortriptyline (Aventyl), and protriptyline (Vivactil).

Definition: Inhibit serotonin and norepinephrine; used to treat both depression and anxiety.

Contraindications: Patients taking MAOIs or other antipsychotics should use caution when taking TCAs. These drugs can alter the effects of antihypertensive, antihistamine, and over-the-counter medications.

Pharmacokinetics: Given orally with food to decrease GI upset.

Side Effects: Anticholinergic effects such as dry mouth, blurry vision, dry mucous membranes, urinary retention, constipation, and change in temperature. Other symptoms are irregular heartbeat, restlessness, change in weight, hypotension, and sexual dysfunction.

Nursing Care: Instruct the patient to take medication as directed. Assess for side effects and treat individually if needed. Advise patients to take tricyclic antidepressants at night to avoid dizziness and sedation. Renal and liver function tests are needed with long-term usage. Assess for suicidal tendencies; a change in behavior can be a clue to these thoughts. Patients who take TCAs are gradually tapered off the medication to avoid discontinuation syndrome, which resembles flulike symptoms.

Monoamine Oxidase Inhibitors (MAOIs)

Types: Phenelzine (Nardil), tranylcypromine (Parnate), moclobemide (Manerix), isocarboxazid (Marplan), and selegiline (Emsam).

Definition: Used if other antidepressants are ineffective. MAOIs inhibit monoamine oxidase, which results in an increase of serotonin and norepinephrine, decreasing symptoms of depression.

Contraindications: MAOIs are contraindicated with many medications and can cause a serious complication known as hypertensive crisis.

Pharmacokinetics: Given orally with food to decrease GI upset. Emsam is given transdermally.

Side Effects: Hypertensive crisis occurs when MAOIs are taken with other medications such as amphetamines, nasal decongestants, opioids, or tyramine. Symptoms of a hypertensive crisis are increased blood pressure, fever, nausea and vomiting, increased heart rate, headache, chest pain, neck stiffness, dilated pupils, and sweating. A hypertensive crisis is treated with phentolamine (Regitine), which is given IV.

Common symptoms of MAOIs are GI upset, anticholinergic symptoms, orthostatic hypotension, dizziness, difficulty sleeping, weight gain, and restlessness.

Nursing Care: Teach patients to take medications as directed. Obtain a medication history in view of the many contraindications, and monitor signs of hypertensive crisis. Monitor blood pressure. Teach the patient to avoid foods with tyramine, such as bananas, cheese, wine, yogurt, figs, raisins, coffee, and certain meats. Patients should use caution when changing position due to the decrease in blood pressure.

Mood Stabilizers

Types of Mood Stabilizers: Lithium, valproate (Depakote), lamotrigine (Lamictal), quetiapine (Seroquel), risperidone (Risperdal), gabapentin (Neurontin), aripiprazole (Abilify), carbamazepine (Tegretol), and olanzapine (Zyprexa).

Definition: Mood stabilizers are given to control manic and depressive episodes in the bipolar patient. Mood stabilizers are often given along with antidepressants. Lithium is the most common medication prescribed for this disorder.

Contraindications: Patients who take MAOIs, diuretics, NSAIDs, or other CNS depressants should use caution when taking mood stabilizers, especially lithium.

Pharmacokinetics: Given orally with food to decrease GI upset.

Side Effects: Lithium, the most common mood stabilizer, can cause toxic symptoms if not taken as directed. Signs of lithium toxicity can vary upon with severity. Symptoms are GI upset, polyuria, polydipsia, sedation, hand tremors, confusion, rigid muscle movements, blurred vision, ringing in the ears, fatigue, and weakness.

Nursing Care: Instruct patients to take medication as directed. Teach the patient to avoid diuretics, caffeine, alcohol, over-the-counter medications, and MAOIs while taking lithium. If not monitored closely, lithium toxicity can occur; these symptoms need to be reported immediately. The therapeutic serum level of lithium is 0.8 to 1.2 mEq/L and is monitored throughout drug therapy. Monitor fluid intake while this medication is being taken. Monitor renal, liver, and cardiac function periodically. Mood stabilizers should not be stopped abruptly but gradually decreased. Patients are monitored for suicidal thoughts or activities throughout the course of therapy.

Cognitive Enhancers

Types: Tacrine (Cognex), donepezil (Aricept), rivastigmine (Exelon), memantine (Namenda), and galantamine (Razadyne).

Definition: These medications inhibit cholinesterase to improve cognition in the Alzheimer's and dementia patient.

Contraindications: Patients with renal and liver disease should use caution when taking these medications. Alzheimer medications can also affect patients with asthma-related ailments and can exacerbate symptoms.

Pharmacokinetics: Given orally with food to decrease GI upset.

Side Effects: Nausea, vomiting, diarrhea, dizziness, weight loss, loss of appetite, constipation, and headache.

Nursing Care: Instruct patients to take medication as directed. Discuss with the patient's family the possibility of their administering the medication if the patient is mentally not capable. Teach the patient/family side effects of the medications and to take with food to avoid GI upset. Renal and liver function tests are assessed periodically throughout therapy. Patients with asthma should use caution when taking these medications because of the potential serious complication of bronchoconstriction.

Advise that these medications only slow the progress of the illness; they do not reverse symptoms. Refer the family for supportive therapy. The patient should keep physically, socially, and mentally active to maximize functioning. Maintain a safe environment.

DECREASING TEST ANXIETY

Sweaty armpits, clammy hands, feeling of impending doom, and feeling like the room is closing in on you are all symptoms of anxiety about taking a nursing test. Many students experience these feelings during a test, and they tend to be overwhelming. The thoughts that run through your head are, "I need to pass this," "I cannot take this class over again," and "I should have studied a little more." You are not alone; many nursing students have the same thoughts. In this chapter, I will talk about ways to decrease anxiety and share some test-taking strategies to help you through both the NCLEX and nursing school. Let's discuss ways to decrease anxiety while test taking.

1. Study! Take your time to learn all the information. Try to study the material every week until the exam. Do not cram! We all do it, but it only increases your anxiety.
2. Attend study groups. Study groups give you not only extra credit but also a better idea of what is on the exam.
3. During your downtime, do something to take your mind off nursing. Relax, eat, see a movie, or just hang out with friends. The downtime will give you a chance to regroup.
4. Positivity! It works. Do not fill your head with negative thoughts. Saying "I'm going to fail" and "I will never pass" is not going to teach you—it will just bring you down. Stay positive. If you study and understand the material, you will be well prepared to pass the exam.
5. Do not stay up all night before exams. Get a good night's rest. This means no partying the night before the exam!
6. Never take a test without eating a good breakfast.
7. Make yourself known to the professor. Meet the professor during office hours. Ask for extra help. This will show the professor you are trying your best.
8. A bad grade on one exam is not going to ruin your nursing career!
9. Buy the recommended study guide. Professors often use the questions in this study guide on the exams.
10. You can do this! I am your cheerleader, rooting for you!

WHAT TO EXPECT IN NURSING SCHOOL

Wouldn't it be great if someone could tell you what to expect in nursing school. The biggest fears are the exams and clinical, the two factors that pretty much make up nursing school. In this book, I have highlighted the most frequently tested information. No, I could not include every single thing, but I have tried to cover all the most important courses. But now I share some more secrets with you. As a former nursing student, I can tell you the ins and outs of how to get through the program.

- Buy the NCLEX book and study guide recommended by the professor; they often use test questions from these books.
- Professors have to have the mean face. It is just what they do. Do not take it personally.
- It really does not matter where you sit. Just as long as you pass.
- Try to make it to clinical on time! You will have points deducted for showing up late.
- Use the PowerPoints as your class notes. There is no need to rewrite what is already written for you.
- Figure out a study method that works for you. The sooner you do this, the better!
- The nurses at clinical are not always happy to see you! Brush it off your shoulders—you are not there to make them happy.
- Try to watch every procedure, insert every IV, and administer medications whenever it is possible.
- Care plans are long, but doing them is part of your clinical grade, so try to finish them as soon as possible.
- Try to stay healthy and fit. Nursing school is exhausting, and staying healthy may help you keep up your energy level.
- You will meet some of your best friends in nursing school!
- Choose a med–surg preceptor; this will give you an idea of what to expect as a nurse. You will figure out whether you want to run or stay.
- You will cry, laugh, and feel helpless at times; that is what nursing is all about!

NCLEX TIPS

1. Practice, practice, practice. Buy an NCLEX book as soon as possible, and start reading the material. Practice the NCLEX questions. This will help you prepare for the exam.
2. Do not wait until the last minute to begin studying. Take the review course offered by your institution, and begin studying soon after graduation.
3. Get more than one study guide with practice CDs. Buy several or exchange with friends; the more questions you answer, the better.
4. Before reserving a date to take the exam, it is best to score 80% or higher on the practice exams. This will better prepare you for the NCLEX and the format of the exam.
5. Come up with a study schedule. Remember to take breaks frequently—attempting to absorb all the information at once can be overwhelming. Take each chapter one at a time, and focus on the material you don't understand.
6. The day before the exam, try to relax and do not study. Take the time to do something fun or enjoyable.
7. The day of the exam eat a proper breakfast. Arrive at the test center early. Arriving late can forfeit your opportunity to take the exam.
8. After the exam, you are going to find yourself in a state of anxiety whether you passed or not. The test is already submitted, and there isn't much that you can do, so relax and wait for the results.
9. If you do not pass the first time, it can be devastating. Take a couple of weeks off. Then begin studying again. Do not schedule a new test date until you are receiving scores of 80% or better on the practice exams.
10. Last but not least, remember that you have completed the nursing program, which means you have already achieved a success. The NCLEX is just another step on the way to your main goal. Stay confident and, before you know it, you will be working on a nursing unit.

ELEVEN

CONCLUSION

Congratulations! You made it to the end. Give yourself a huge pat on the back. You have worked hard, studied hard, and put lots of time into completing the nursing program. Yes, there was a ton of information in this book, and your head may be spinning. Take each course one at a time. This book is designed to be used as a study guide alongside your textbook and class notes. As you have completed this book, you will have noticed that only the most important information is conveyed, with information for you to concentrate on highlighted. Use this book throughout your nursing education; this is a guideline for you to follow. I am proud to bring you this book and share these tips with you.

You are so close to graduating and becoming a nurse. The NCLEX is the next step to becoming an RN. First, enjoy the moment when you graduate from nursing school. You have worked so hard for this moment. Enjoy it, take it all in, and go celebrate! Take a week to relax and kick back before you start studying for the NCLEX.

Completing nursing school and the NCLEX brings you to another major pinnacle of your nursing career. Be proud to carry RN next to your name—you worked very hard for the title. As you enter your first nursing job, you will notice quickly the series of emotions you will go through. Emotions such as anxiety, nervousness, fear, confusion, and a little excitement were the feelings I felt during the first days of my nursing career. These emotions slowly dissipate as you become more comfortable with the task at hand. Six years into my career as a nurse, I realized that it is impossible to know everything in the nursing field. Nursing is a field in which education is ongoing. There are always new medications and ailments that you will be responsible for knowing. At times it is challenging, but it is a very rewarding and humbling career. I am proud to be a nurse and always will be. I will be forever grateful for the opportunities to touch people's lives.

ABBREVIATIONS

ABG	arterial blood gas (test)
ADH	antidiuretic hormone
ADL	activities of daily living
ALT	alanine aminotransferase
AST	aspartate aminotransferase
BBB	blood–brain barrier
BP	blood pressure
bpm	beats per minute
BUN	blood urea nitrogen
Ca	calcium
CAD	coronary artery disease
CBC	complete blood count
CF	cystic fibrosis
CHF	congestive heart failure
CK	creatine kinase
CNS	central nervous system
cpm	cycles per minute
CSF	cerebral spinal fluid
CT	computed tomography
CVS	chorionic villus sampling
DVT	deep vein thrombosis
EEG	electroencephalogram
EIA	enzyme immunoassay (test)
EKG	electrocardiogram
ELISA	enzyme-linked immunosorbent assay
FHR	fetal heart rate
GERD	gastroesophageal reflux disease
GH	growth hormone
GI	gastrointestinal
H&H	hematocrit and hemoglobin
HA	headache
Hgb	hemoglobin
HOB	head of bed
HTN	hypertension
I/O	intake/output

ICP	intracranial pressure
ICU	intensive care unit
IFA	immunofluorescence assay
IM	intramuscular
IVF	intravenous fluids
IVIg	intravenous immunoglobulin
K	potassium
LFT	liver function test
LGA	large for gestational age
LTB	laryngotracheobronchitis; "croup"
LUQ	left upper quadrant
MAOI	monoamine oxidase inhibitor
MI	myocardial infarction
MRI	magnetic resonance imaging
MRSA	methicillin-resistant Staphylococcus aureus
N/V/D	nausea, vomiting, diarrhea
NCLEX	National Council Licensure Examination
NGT	nasogastric tube
NSAIDs	nonsteroidal anti-inflammatory drugs
O_2	oxygen
PFT	pulmonary function test
PO	*per os*; "orally"
PPD	positive purified protein derivative
PT/INR	prothrombin time and international normalized ratio
PTT	partial thromboplastin time
RhoGAM	Rho(D) immune globulin
RLQ	right lower quadrant
ROM	range of motion
RSV	respiratory syncytial virus
SA node	sinoatrial node
SNRI	serotonin and norepinephrine reuptake inhibitor
SOB	side of bed
SQ	subcutaneously
STI	sexually transmitted infection
TB	tuberculosis
TCA	tricyclic antidepressants
TEF	tracheoesophageal fistula
UTI	urinary tract infection
WBC	white blood cell (count)

NCLEX QUESTION FORMATS

To pass the NCLEX-RN® examination, you will have to answer a minimum of 60 questions at the set competency level. Some students can accomplish this in 75 questions (60 at the set competency level plus 15 pretest questions). If you answer 265 questions, a final ability estimate is computed to determine if you are successful. If you run out of time and have not completed all 265 questions, you can still pass if you have answered the last 60 questions at the set competency level. Approximately 1.3 minutes are allocated for each question, but we all know that some questions take a short time to answer, while others, including math questions, may take longer.

The NCLEX-RN exam now comprises several different types of questions, including hot spots, fill-in-the-blank, drag-and-drop, order-response, and select-all-that-apply or multiple-response questions. These are referred to as alternative types of questions and have been added to better assess your critical thinking. This book offers plenty of practice with such questions. Examples of the *select-all-that-apply* type of question are shown in Exercises 1 and 2.

Exercise 1

Select all that apply:
The nurse is reviewing data collected from a patient who is being treated for hypothyroidism. Which information indicates that the patient has had a positive outcome?

A. Sleeps 8 hours each night, waking up to go to the bathroom once.
B. Has bowel movements two times a week while on a high-fiber diet.

From Wittmann-Price, R. A., & Thompson, B. R. (Eds.). (2010). *NCLEX-RN® EXCEL: Test through unfolding case study review* (pp. 7–12, 20–24). New York, NY: Springer Publishing.

C. Gained 10 pounds since the initial clinic visit 6 weeks ago.
D. Was promoted at work because of increased work production.
E. Walks 2 miles within 30 minutes before work each morning.

The answer can be found on page 273

Exercise 2

Select all that apply:
The hospital is expecting to receive survivors of a disaster. The charge nurse is directed to provide a list of patients for possible discharge. Which of the following patients would be placed on the list?

A. A patient who was admitted 3 days ago with urosepsis; white blood cell count is 5.4 $mm^3/\mu L$.
B. A patient who was admitted 2 days ago after an acetaminophen overdose; creatinine is 2.1 mg/dL.
C. A patient who was admitted with stable angina and had two stents placed in the left anterior descending coronary artery 24 hours ago.
D. A patient who was admitted with an upper gastrointestinal bleed and had an endoscopic ablation 48 hours ago; hemoglobin is 10.8 g/dL.

The answer can be found on page 274

An example of an NCLEX-RN *fill-in-the-blank* question is provided in Exercise 3.

Exercise 3

Fill in the blanks:
The nurse is calculating the client's total intake and output to determine whether he has a positive or negative fluid balance. The intake includes the following:

1,200 mL IV D5NSS

200 mL of vancomycin IV

Two 8-ounce glasses of juice

One 4-ounce cup of broth

One 6-ounce cup of water

Upon being emptied, the Foley bag was found to contain 350 mL of urine. What would the nurse document?

The answer can be found on page 274

Drag-and-drop questions are specific to the computer because the student uses a mouse or touch pad to place items in order. A hot spot is moving the mouse or the touch plate to a specific point on a diagram. An example of an NCLEX-RN hot-spot question is provided in Exercise 4.

Exercise 4

Hot spot:
The nurse assesses a patient who has a possible brain tumor. The patient has difficulty coordinating voluntary muscle movement and balance. Which area of the brain is affected? (Please place an X at the appropriate spot.)

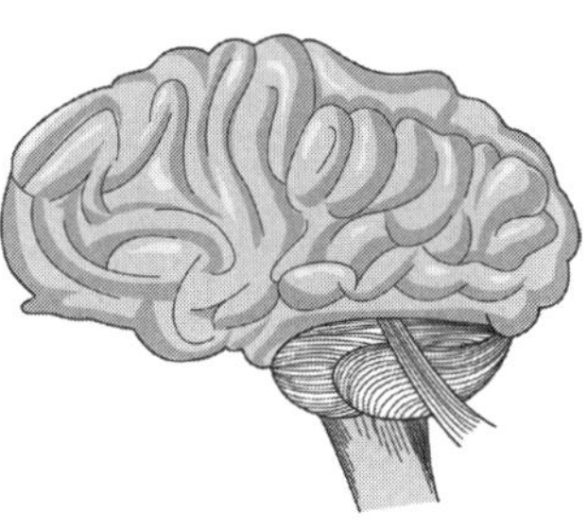

The answer can be found on page 275

An example of an *ordering* NCLEX-RN question is found in Exercise 5.

Exercise 5

Ordering:
The nurse is inserting an indwelling urinary catheter into a female patient. Place the steps in the correct order:

____ Ask the patient to bear down.
____ Don clean gloves, and wash the perineal area.
____ Place the client in a dorsal recumbent position.
____ Advance the catheter 1.2 inches (2.5 to 5 cm).
____ Inflate the balloon and pull back gently.

____ Retract the labia with the nondominant hand.
____ Use forceps with the dominant hand to cleanse the perineal area.
____ Place drapes on the bed and over the perineal area.
____ Apply sterile gloves.
____ Advance the catheter 2 to 3 inches (5 to 7 cm) until urine drains.
____ Test balloon, lubricate catheter, place antiseptic on cotton balls.

The answer can be found on page 275

An example of an NCLEX-RN *exhibit-format* question is provided in Exercise 6.

Exercise 6

Exhibit-format question:
A 52-year-old female patient admitted to the emergency department (ED) has had nausea and vomiting for 3 days and abdominal pain that is unrelieved after vomiting.

Skin: Pale, cool; patient shivering.

Respiration: RR 30, lungs clear, SaO_2 90.

CV: RRR (regular rate and rhythm) with mitral regurgitation; temperature 95°F (35°C), BP 96/60, pulse 132 and weak.

Extremities: + 4 pulses, no edema of lower extremities.

GI: Hyperactive bowel sounds; vomited 100 mL of bile-colored fluid, positive abdominal tenderness.

GU: Foley inserted, no urine drained.

- Hemoglobin 10.6 g/dL
- Hematocrit 39%
- White blood cells 8.0 mm^3/µL
- Sodium 150 mEq/L
- Potassium 7.0 mEq/L
- Blood urea nitrogen 132 mg/dL
- Creatinine 8.2 mg/dL
- Serum amylase 972
- Serum lipase 1,380
- Arterial blood gas pH 7.0

- pO_2 90 mmHg
- pCO_2 39 mmHg
- HCO_3 17 mEq/L

After reviewing the patient's assessment findings and laboratory reports, the nurse determines that the priority for the plan of care should focus on:

A. Metabolic acidosis and oliguria
B. Respiratory acidosis and dyspnea
C. Metabolic alkalosis related to vomiting
D. Respiratory alkalosis resulting from abdominal pain

The answer can be found on page 276

Another strategy to use in studying for the NCLEX-RN exam is to become familiar with the organization of the test. The test plan covers the four basic categories of client needs, including safe and effective care environment, health promotion and maintenance, psychosocial integrity, and physiological integrity. The following questions are designed to test your grasp of providing a "safe and effective environment" through the way you manage patient care, which is an important aspect of your role and responsibility as a licensed RN. This concept applies to what you should do as an RN as well as the tasks you can delegate to nonlicensed personnel working with you. Exercises 7 and 8 offer examples of questions based on the RN's responsibility for managing safe and effective patient care.

Exercise 7

Multiple-choice question:
After returning from a hip replacement, a patient with diabetes mellitus type 1 is lethargic, flushed, and feeling nauseated. Vital signs are BP 108/78, P 100, R 24 and deep. What is the next action the nurse should take?

A. Notify the physician.
B. Check the patient's glucose.
C. Administer an antiemetic.
D. Change the IV infusion rate.

The answer can be found on page 277

Exercise 8

Multiple-choice question:
The nurse is assigned to care for a patient with pneumonia. Which task can be delegated to the unlicensed assistive personnel by the RN?

A. Teaching a patient how to use the inhaler.
B. Listening to the patient's lungs.
C. Checking the results of the patient's blood work.
D. Counting the patient's respiratory rate.

The answer can be found on page 277

Yet another strategy to use in analyzing NCLEX-RN questions is to assess the negative/positive balance of the question. For a positive question, select the option that is correct; for a negative question, select the option that is incorrect. Examples of NCLEX-RN questions with positive and negative answers are shown in Table 1.

TABLE 1

Positive NCLEX-RN type of question stem	Negative NCLEX-RN type of question stem
Which statement by the client *indicates an understanding* of the medication side effects?	Which statement by the client *indicates a need for further teaching* about the medication side effects?

Therapeutic communication is one of the long-enduring basics of nursing care. As RNs, we provide therapy, not only through what we do but also through what and how we communicate with patients and families. Therapeutic communication is not what you would use in everyday conversation, because it is designed to be more purposeful. Therapeutic communication is nonjudgmental, direct, truthful, empathetic, and informative. Communication and documentation are among the important threads integrated throughout the NCLEX-RN examination. An example of an NCLEX-RN question based on therapeutic communication is shown in Exercise 9.

Exercise 9

Multiple-choice question:
An 11-year-old boy with acute lymphocytic leukemia (ALL) has been diagnosed with his second relapse following successful remissions after chemotherapy and radiation. The patient asks, "Am I going to die?" Which response by the nurse would be most helpful to the patient?

A. "Let's talk about this after I speak with your parents."
B. "Can you tell me why you feel this way?"
C. "You will need to discuss this with the oncologist."
D. "You sound like you'd like to talk about it."

The answer can be found on page 277

ANSWERS

Exercise 1

Select all that apply:
The nurse is reviewing data collected from a patient who is being treated for hypothyroidism. Which information indicates that the patient has had a positive outcome?

A. Sleeps 8 hours each night, waking up to go to the bathroom once. YES; hypothyroidism causes severe fatigue; 8 hours of sleep and waking up once are normal.
B. Has bowel movements two times a week while on a high-fiber diet. NO; this may be constipation.
C. Gained 10 pounds since the initial clinic visit 6 weeks ago. NO; this is not an expected outcome.
D. Was promoted at work because of increased work production. YES; energy levels are expected to increase.
E. Walks 2 miles within 30 minutes before work each morning. YES; energy levels are expected to increase.

Exercise 2

Select all that apply:

The hospital is expecting to receive survivors of a disaster. The charge nurse is directed to provide a list of patients for possible discharge. Which of the following patients would be placed on the list?

A. A patient who was admitted 3 days ago with urosepsis; white blood cell count is 5.4 $mm^3/\mu L$. YES; this patient has a normal WBC count and could be discharged.
B. A patient who was admitted 2 days ago after an acetaminophen overdose; creatinine is 2.1 mg/dL. NO; this patient has a high creatinine level and needs monitoring.
C. A patient who was admitted with stable angina and had two stents placed in the left anterior descending coronary artery 24 hours ago. YES; patients who have not had an MI (myocardial infarction) but have had stents normally are discharged in 24 hours.
D. A patient who was admitted with an upper gastrointestinal bleed and had an endoscopic ablation 48 hours ago; hemoglobin is 10.8 g/dL. YES; the patient has no active bleeding, and the hemoglobin is stable.

Exercise 3

Fill in the blanks:

The nurse is calculating the client's total intake and output to determine whether he has a positive or negative fluid balance. The intake includes the following:

1,200 mL IV D5NSS

200 mL vancomycin IV

Two 8-ounce glasses of juice

One 4-ounce cup of broth

One 6-ounce cup of water

Upon being emptied, the Foley bag was found to contain 350 mL of urine. What would the nurse document?

Total intake: 2,180 mL

Total output: –350 mL

Positive fluid balance: 1,830 mL

Exercise 4

Hot spot:
The nurse assesses a patient who has a possible brain tumor. The patient has difficulty coordinating voluntary muscle movement and balance. Which area of the brain is affected? (Please place an X at the appropriate spot.)

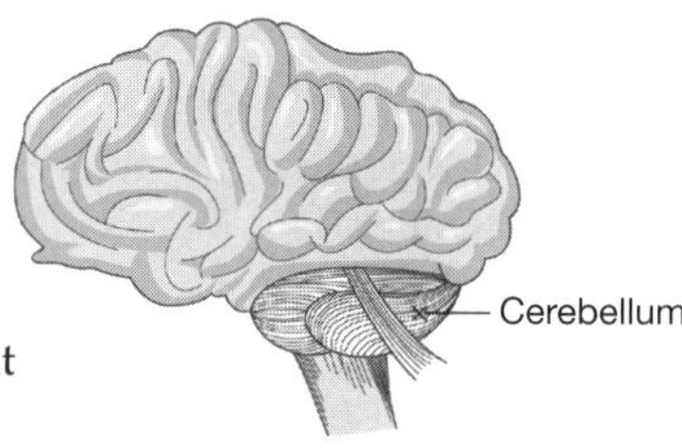

Exercise 5

Ordering:
The nurse is inserting an indwelling urinary catheter into a female patient. Place the steps in the correct order:

8. Ask the patient to bear down.
2. Don clean gloves, and wash the perineal area.
1. Place the client in a dorsal recumbent position.
10. Advance the catheter 1.2 inches (2.5 to 5 cm).
11. Inflate the balloon and pull back gently.
6. Retract the labia with the nondominant hand.
7. Use forceps with the dominant hand to cleanse the perineal area.
3. Place drapes on the bed and over the perineal area.
4. Apply sterile gloves.
9. Advance the catheter 2 to 3 inches (5 to 7 cm) until urine drains.
5. Test balloon, lubricate catheter, place antiseptic on cotton balls.

The sterile gloves are usually packaged under the drapes. Therefore, the drapes can be appropriately placed to set up a sterile field and drape the patient by touching their outer corners. The gloves are usually donned after the drapes are in place. It is not incorrect to place sterile gloves on prior to draping.

Exercise 6

Exhibit-format question:

A 52-year-old female patient admitted to the emergency department (ED) has had nausea and vomiting for 3 days and abdominal pain that is unrelieved after vomiting.

Skin: Pale, cool; patient shivering.

Respiration: RR 30, lungs clear, SaO_2 90.

CV: RRR (regular rate and rhythm) with mitral regurgitation; temperature 95°F (35°C), BP 96/60, pulse 132 and weak.

Extremities: + 4 pulses, no edema of lower extremities.

GI: Hyperactive bowel sounds; vomited 100 mL of bile-colored fluid, positive abdominal tenderness.

GU: Foley inserted, no urine drained.

- Hemoglobin 10.6 g/dL
- Hematocrit 39%
- White blood cells 8.0 $mm^3/\mu L$
- Sodium 150 mEq/L
- Potassium 7.0 mEq/L
- Blood urea nitrogen 132 mg/dL
- Creatinine 8.2 mg/dL
- Serum amylase 972
- Serum lipase 1,380
- Arterial blood gas pH 7.0
- pO_2 90 mmHg
- pCO_2 39 mmHg
- HCO_3 17 mEq/L

After reviewing the patient's assessment findings and laboratory reports, the nurse determines that the priority for the plan of care should focus on:

A. Metabolic acidosis and oliguria. YES; the pH and HCO_3 are decreased, and the patient has no urine output.
B. Respiratory acidosis and dyspnea. NO; the lungs are clear, and there is no other indication of respiratory acidosis.
C. Metabolic alkalosis related to vomiting. NO; the pH is low.
D. Respiratory alkalosis resulting from abdominal pain. NO; the pH is low, and the pCO_2 is normal.

Exercise 7

Multiple-choice question:
After returning from a hip replacement, a patient with diabetes mellitus type 1 is lethargic, flushed, and feeling nauseated. Vital signs are BP 108/78, P 100, R 24 and deep. What is the next action the nurse should take?

A. Notify the physician. NO; the nurse needs to further assess.
B. Check the patient's glucose. YES; these are signs of hypoglycemia.
C. Administer an antiemetic. NO; this will not help.
D. Change the IV infusion rate. NO; this will not help.

Exercise 8

Multiple-choice question:
The nurse is assigned to care for a patient with pneumonia. Which task can be delegated to the unlicensed assistive personnel by the RN?

A. Teaching a patient how to use the inhaler. NO; an RN must do initial patient teaching.
B. Listening to the patient's lungs. NO; an RN must do an initial assessment.
C. Checking the results of the patient's blood work. NO; an RN must interpret lab results.
D. Counting the patient's respiratory rate. YES; unlicensed personnel can obtain vital signs.

Exercise 9

Multiple-choice question:
An 11-year-old boy with acute lymphocytic leukemia (ALL) has been diagnosed with his second relapse following successful remissions after chemotherapy and radiation. The patient asks, "Am I going to die?" Which response by the nurse would be most helpful to the patient?

A. "Let's talk about this after I speak with your parents." NO; this is not responding to the patient.
B. "Can you tell me why you feel this way?" NO; although this is not a completely wrong answer, it is more directive and may intimidate a child.
C. "You will need to discuss this with the oncologist." NO; this is not responding to the patient's question and is not at his developmental level.
D. "You sound like you'd like to talk about it." YES; this is using probing to help the patient to dialogue.

BASIC EKG RHYTHM EXAMPLES

Sinus Rhythm

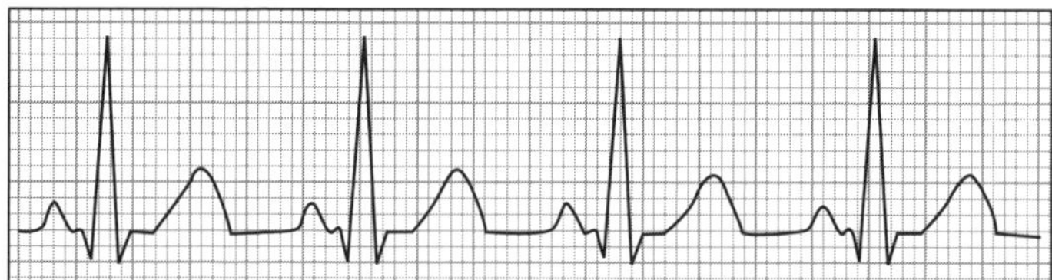

Sinus Bradycardia

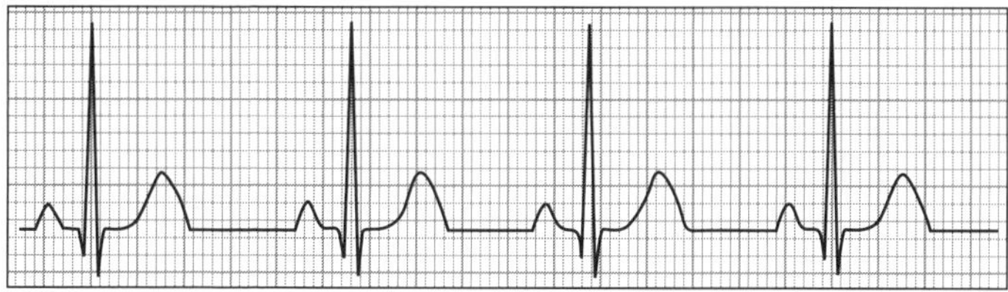

Sinus Tachycardia

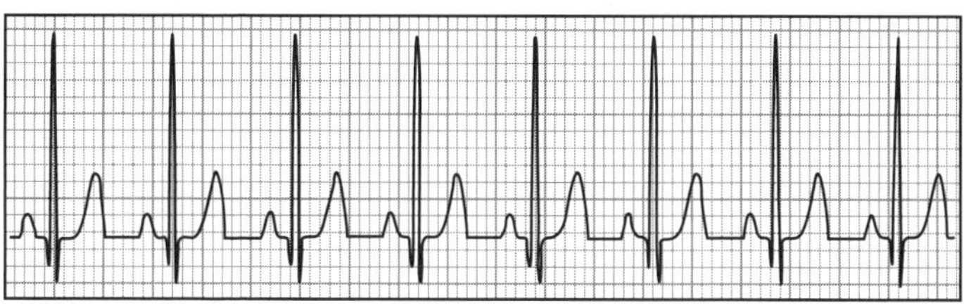

First-Degree Heart Block

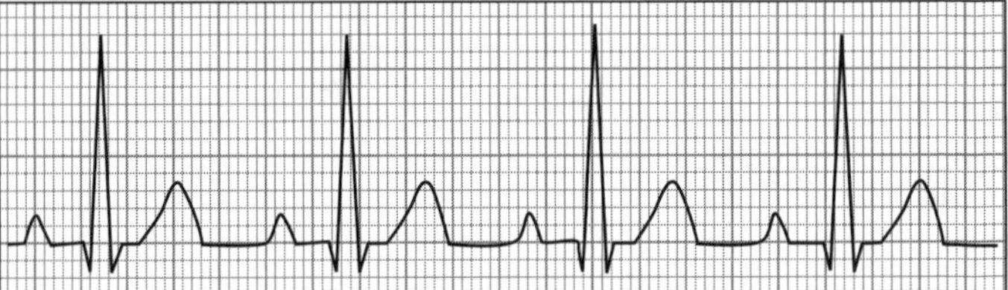

Second-Degree Heart Block, Type I Wenckebach

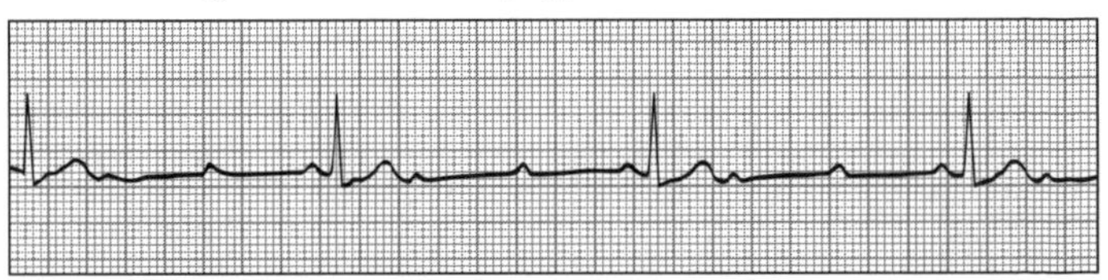

Second-Degree Heart Block, Type II

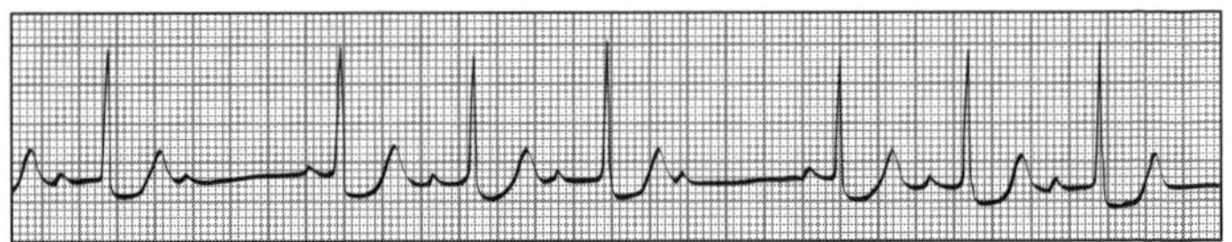

Third-Degree Heart Block

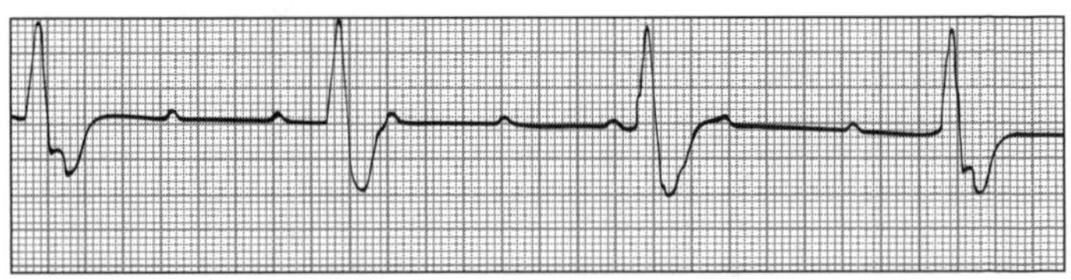

Atrial Flutter

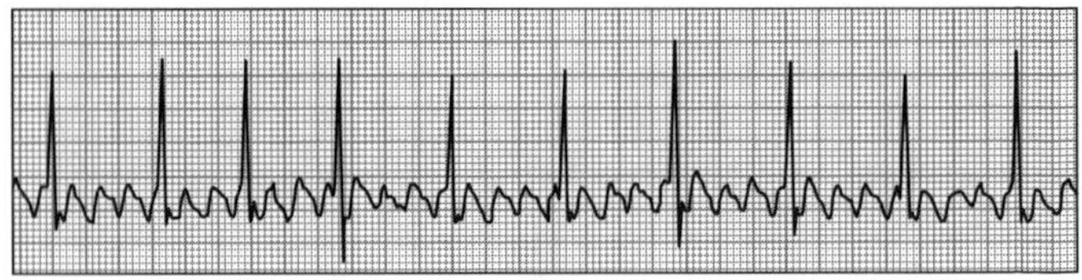

Atrial Fibrillation

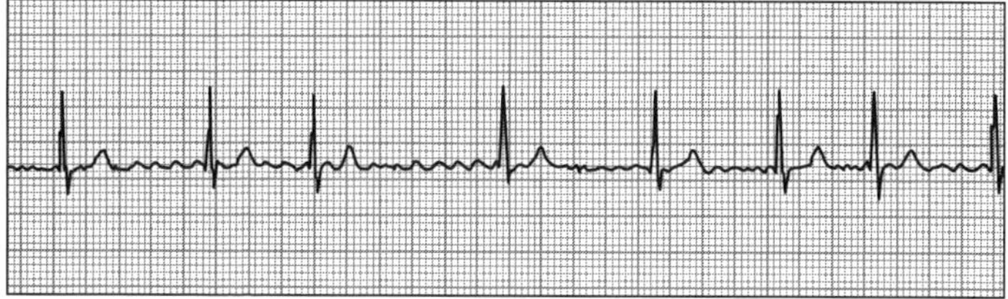

Junctional

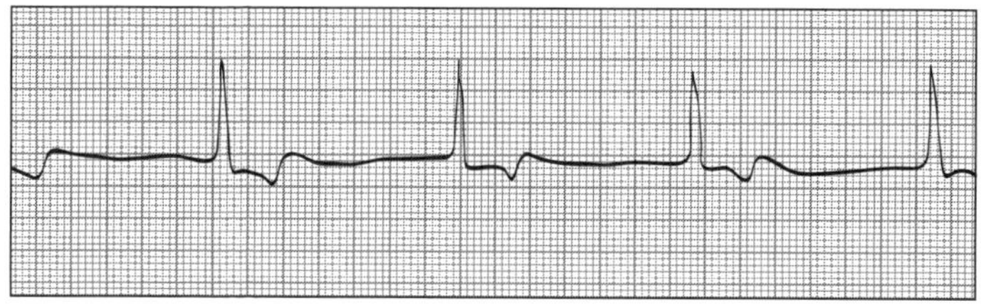

Supraventricular Tachycardia

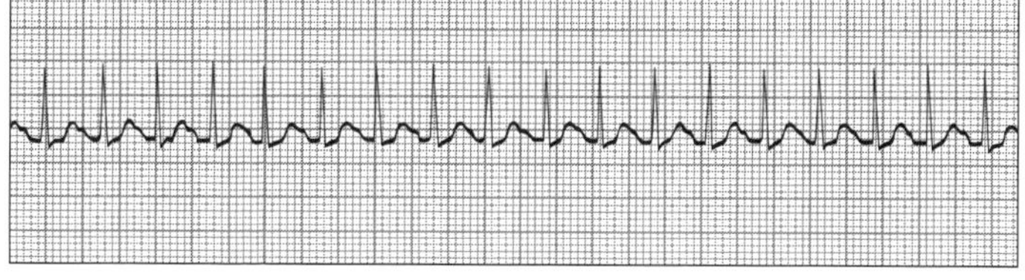

Paroxysmal Supraventricular Tachycardia

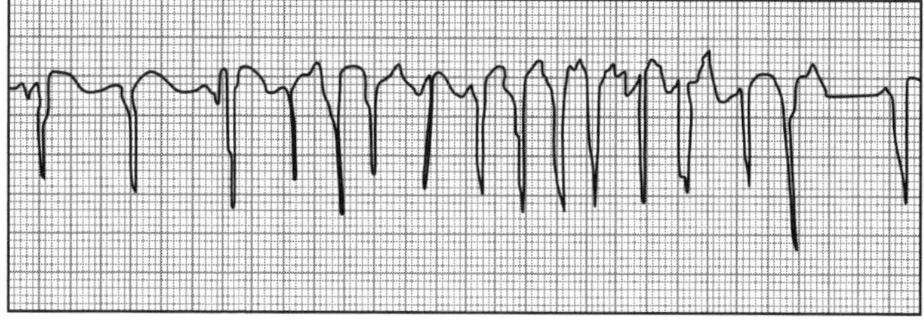

Idioventricular

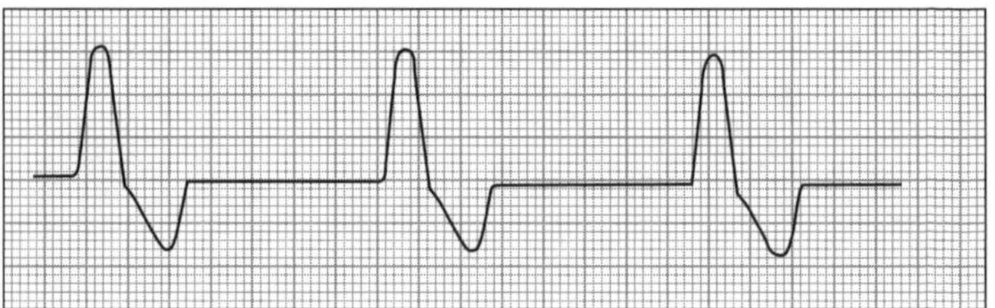

Sinus Rhythm With Unifocal PVCs

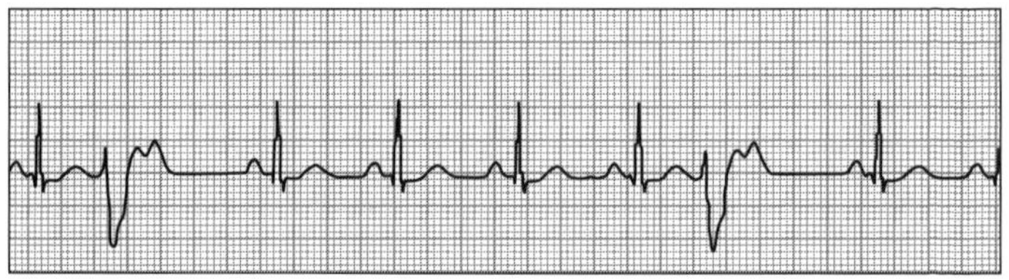

Sinus Rhythm With Multifocal PVCs

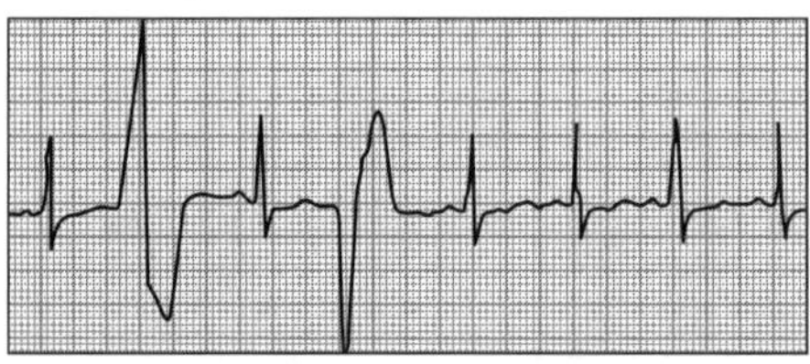

Bigeminal PVCs

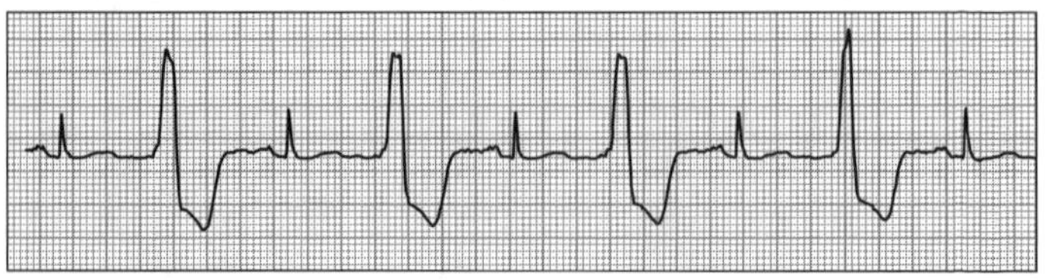

Ventricular Tachycardia

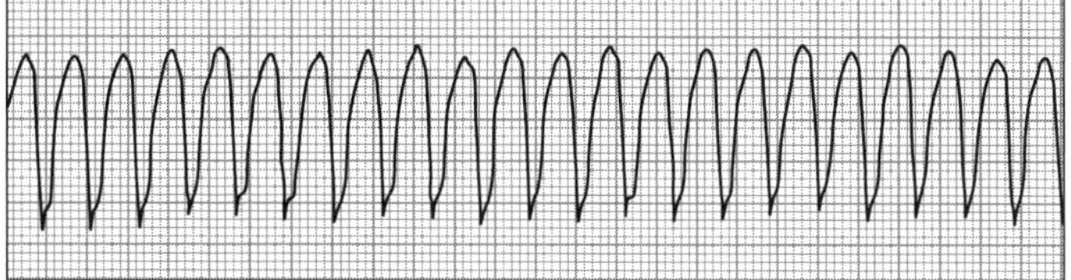

Ventricular Fibrillation

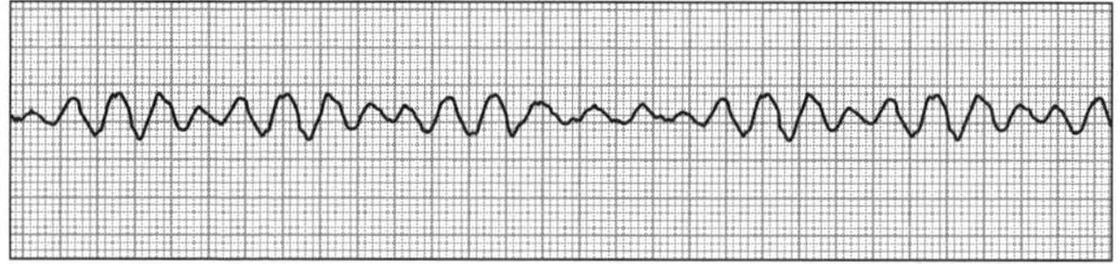

Ventricular Pacing

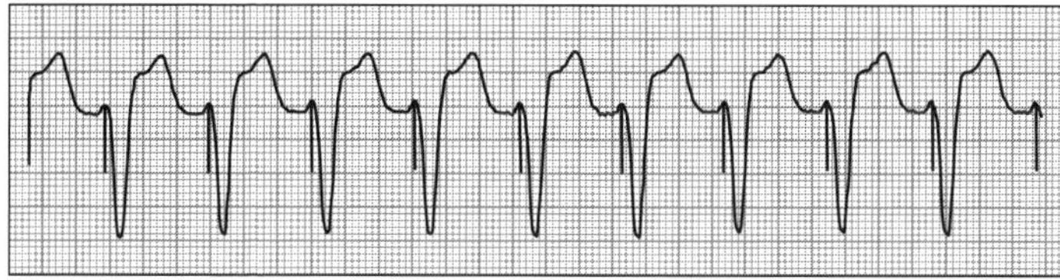

Asystole

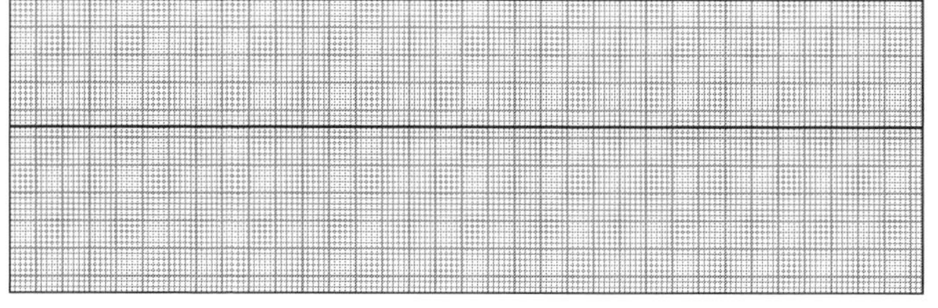

BIBLIOGRAPHY

Berman, A. T., & Snyder, S. (2011). *Kozier & Erb's Fundamentals of nursing: Concepts, process, and practice* (9th ed.). Upper Saddle River, NJ: Prentice-Hall.

Davidson, M., London, M., & Ladewig, P. W. (2011). *Old's maternal–newborn nursing and women's health across the lifespan* (9th ed.). Upper Saddle River, NJ: Prentice Hall.

Hockenberry, M. J., & Wilson, D. (2012). *Wong's essentials of pediatric nursing* (9th ed.). St. Louis, MO: Mosby.

Jarvis, C. (2011). *Physical examination and health assessment* (6th ed.). St. Louis, MO: Saunders Elsevier.

Lehne, R. (2010). *Pharmacology for nursing care* (7th ed.). St. Louis, MO: Saunders Elsevier.

Lewis, S., Dirksen, S., Heitkemper, M., & Bucher., L. (2013). *Medical-surgical nursing: Assessment and management of clinical problems* (9th ed.). St Louis, MO: Mosby.

Lewis, S., Heitkemper, M., & Dirksen, S. (2011). *Medical–surgical nursing: Assessment and management of clinical problem* (8th ed.). St. Louis, MO: Mosby.

Potter, A. Perry, A., Stockert P., & Hall, A. (2013) *Fundamentals of nursing* (8th ed.). St. Louis, MO: Mosby.

INDEX